Topics in Neuroscience

Managing Editor:

GIANCARLO COMI

Co-Editor:

JACOPO MELDOLESI

Associate Editors:

UGO ECARI

MASSIMO FILIPPI

GIANVITO MARTINO

Springer

Milano
Berlin
Heidelberg
New York
Barcelona
Hong Kong
London
Paris
Singapore
Tokyo

M. Filippi • G. Comi (Eds)

Primary Progressive Multiple Sclerosis

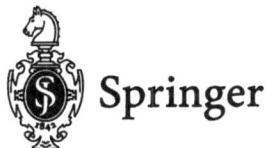 Springer

MASSIMO FILIPPI
Neuroimaging Research Unit
Department of Neuroscience
Scientific Institute and University
Ospedale San Raffaele, Milan, Italy

GIANCARLO COMI
Clinical Trials Unit
Department of Neuroscience
Scientific Institute and University
Ospedale San Raffaele, Milan, Italy

The Editors and Authors wish to thank FARMADES-SCHERING GROUP (Italy) for the support and help in the realization and promotion of this volume

Springer-Verlag Italia
a member of BertelsmannSpringer Science+Business Media GmbH

© Springer-Verlag Italia, Milano 2002

Softcover reprint of the hardcover 1st edition 2002

http://www.springer.de

ISBN-13: 978-88-470-2236-2   e-ISBN-13: 978-88-470-2234-8
DOI: 10.1007/978-88-470-2234-8

Library of Congress Cataloging-in-Publication Data: applied for

Typesetting: Copy Card Center s.r.l. (Milan)

Cover design: Simona Colombo

SPIN: 10848947

Foreword

"Why are there no effective treatments for my condition? Why do researchers exclude patients with primary progressive multiple sclerosis from enrolling in clinical trials? Please let me know if you hear of studies that I might be allowed to enter or treatments that I could try for my condition."

Thus, in recent years, the sad lament of the patient with primary progressive MS (PPMS). This variant, often in the guise of a chronic progressive myelopathy or, less commonly, progressive cerebellar or bulbar dysfunction, usually responds poorly to corticosteroids and rarely seems to benefit to a significant degree from intensive immunosuppressive treatments. In recent years, most randomized clinical trials have excluded PPMS patients on two counts. Clinical worsening develops slowly in PPMS and may not be recognized during the course of a 2- or 3-year trial even in untreated control patients. This factor alone adds to the potential for a type 2 error or, at the very least, inflates the sample size and duration of the trial. In addition, there is mounting evidence that progressive axonal degeneration and neuronal loss (rather than active, recurrent inflammation) may be important components of the pathology in this form of the disease. Although contemporary trials are evaluating whether PPMS patients may benefit from treatment with the β-interferons and glatiramer acetate, preliminary, uncontrolled clinical experience suggests that the results may not be dramatic.

When faced with a case of possible PPMS, neurologists appropriately focus on making an accurate diagnosis, taking great care to exclude potentially treatable conditions that may have a similar clinical presentation. They then concentrate on patient education, treat complications as these develop, and prescribe physical medicine and rehabilitation measures to enhance quality of life. A few neurologists continue to test whether strategies designed to alter immune function may help, but it seems that enthusiasm for this approach is waning. There is a growing consensus that opportunities to influence the course of the disease may need to await additional insights into the pathogenesis and, perhaps, the development of treatment strategies that will enhance the survival and repair of damaged axons ("neuroprotection and axonal regeneration").

This monograph by Dr. Massimo Filippi and Prof. Giancarlo Comi and their colleagues brings together many of the leading groups in this field to review the considerable progress made in understanding this variant of MS. These reviews clearly demonstrate that the advances in understanding the natural history, pathophysiology, pathogenesis, and pathology of PPMS are being extended by ongoing studies of the MS plaque and normal-appearing white matter using magnetic resonance imaging and spectroscopic techniques. This confluence of thought provides insight into possible disease mechanisms. In short order we can anticipate testable hypotheses, treatment trials with agents resulting from this era of "the new biology" and, hopefully, the end to the sad lament of the person suffering from PPMS.

J.H. Noseworthy, MD
Mayo Clinic
Rochester, MN, USA

Table of Contents

List of Contributors

M.P. Amato
Department of Neurology,
University of Florence, Italy
e-mail: mariapia.amato@unifi.it

D.L. Arnold
Magnetic Resonance Spectroscopy Unit,
Montreal Neurological Institute,
McGill University, Montreal,
Quebec, Canada
e-mail: doug@mrs.mni.mcgill.ca

J. Baskerville
The Multiple Sclerosis Clinic,
University of Western Ontario, London,
Ontario, Canada
e-mail: jbaskerville@sympatico.ca

W. Brück
Department of Neuropathology, Charité,
Campus Virchow-Klinikum, Berlin,
Germany
e-mail: wolfgang.brueck@charite.de

Z. Caramanos
Magnetic Resonance Spectroscopy Unit,
Montreal Neurological Institute,
McGill University, Montreal,
Quebec, Canada
e-mail: aki@mrs.mni.mcgill.ca

G. Comi
Clinical Trials Unit, Department of
Neuroscience, Scientific Institute and
University Ospedale San Raffaele, Milan,
Italy
e-mail: g.comi@hsr.it

D. Cottrell
Department of Neurology,
University of Newcastle-upon-Tyne, UK
e-mail: D.A.Cottrell@newcastle.ac.uk

G. Ebers
Department of Clinical Neurology,
Radcliffe Infirmary, University of Oxford,
Oxford, UK
e-mail: george.ebers@clneuro.ox.ac.uk

M. Filippi
Neuroimaging Research Unit,
Department of Neuroscience,
Scientific Institute and University
Ospedale San Raffaele, Milan, Italy
e-mail: filippi.massimo@hsr.it

S.J. Francis
Magnetic Resonance Spectroscopy Unit,
Montreal Neurological Institute,
McGill University, Montreal,
Quebec, Canada
e-mail: simon@mrs.mni.mcgill.ca

R. He
Department of Radiology,
University of Texas-Houston,
Health Science Center, Houston,
Texas, USA

G.T. Ingle
NMR Research Unit, Institute of
Neurology, Queen Square, London, UK
e-mail: g.ingle@ion.ucl.ac.uk

M. Kremenchutzky
Department of Clinical Neurological
Sciences, London Health Science Centre,
University of Western Ontario, London,
Ontario, Canada
e-mail: mkremenc@uwo.ca

L. Leocani
Neurophysiology Department,
Scientific Institute and University
Ospedale San Raffaele, Milan, Italy
e-mail: l.leocani@hsr.it

D.H. Miller
NMR Research Unit, Institute of
Neurology, Queen Square, London, UK
e-mail: d.miller@ion.ucl.ac.uk

X. Montalban
Hopital General, Unitat de
Neuroimmunologia Clinica,
U.G.U. Vall d'Hebron, Barcelona, Spain
e-mail: xmontal@hg.vhebron.es

P.A. Narayana
Departments of Radiology,
The University of Texas-Houston,
Health Science Center, Houston,
Texas, USA
e-mail: Ponnada.A.Narayana@uth.tmc.edu

S. Narayanan
Magnetic Resonance Spectroscopy Unit,
Montreal Neurological Institute,
McGill University, Montreal,
Quebec, Canada
e-mail: sridar@mrs.mni.mcgill.ca

D. Pelletier
UCSF Multiple Sclerosis Center,
University of California, San Francisco,
California, USA
e-mail: pelletier@mscenter.ucsf.edu

G. Rice
The Multiple Sclerosis Clinic,
University of Western Ontario, London,
Ontario, Canada
e-mail: grice@uwo.ca

M.A. Rocca
Neuroimaging Research Unit,
Department of Neuroscience,
Scientific Institute and University
Ospedale San Raffaele, Milan, Italy
e-mail: mara.rocca@hsr.it

M. Rovaris
Neuroimaging Research Unit,
Department of Neuroscience,
Scientific Institute and University
Ospedale San Raffaele, Milan, Italy
e-mail: rovaris.marco@hsr.it

A.C. Santos
Magnetic Resonance Spectroscopy Unit,
Montreal Neurological Institute,
McGill University, Montreal,
Quebec, Canada
e-mail: santos@mrs.mni.mcgill.ca

A.J. Thompson
NMR Research Unit, Institute of
Neurology, Queen Square, London, UK
e-mail: a.thompson@ion.ucl.ac.uk

J.S. Wolinsky
Department of Neurology, University
of Texas-Houston, Health Science Center,
Houston, Texas, USA
e-mail: jswolinsky@aol.com

Introduction

M. Filippi, M. Rovaris, G. Comi

Since the earliest clinical studies of multiple sclerosis (MS), it has been recognized that a subgroup of patients follows a pattern of disease evolution which is progressive from onset and, as a consequence, has been termed "primary progressive" (PP). Although only 10%-15% of the overall MS patient population is affected by PPMS, this condition on the one hand poses intriguing questions about the nature of the pathophysiological mechanisms underlying the progressive accumulation of neurological disability, and on the other represents an important clinical challenge.

Several pieces of evidence indicate that PPMS has immunopathological characteristics that differ from those of patients with the more "classical" forms of the disease. Since the advent of magnetic resonance imaging (MRI), which enabled us to obtain accurate in vivo estimates of the dynamics of MS activity and evolution, it has been consistently found that, although PPMS patients experience a progressive accumulation of neurological disability from onset, the burden and activity of lesions on conventional MRI scans are on average much lower than in other MS phenotypes. These findings agree with those of histopathological studies, which showed that PPMS lesions are characterized by loss of myelin and axons, with only mild inflammatory components. The paucity of macroscopic lesions in PPMS has resulted in the search for other factors with the potential to cause a progressive accumulation of irreversible neurological disability in these patients. In the last few years, several studies based on nonconventional MR technology have suggested that three factors are likely to contribute to the clinical manifestations of the disease: the presence of diffuse, microscopic damage in the brain tissue which appears normal on conventional MRI scans, a predominant involvement of the spinal cord, and the progressive failure of reparative mechanisms. Although it is still a matter of debate, there is a general feeling in the scientific community (as witness also many of the contributions of this book) that the differences outlined between PPMS and other MS phenotypes are quantitative rather than qualitative. The study of PPMS has, therefore, the potential to increase our understanding of the pathophysiological mechanisms underlying the accumulation of progressive disability in MS in the absence of acute clinical deteriorations and with only a mild inflammatory background.

The difficulty in making a clinical diagnosis of PPMS, as well as the somewhat unsatisfactory way PPMS has been previously classified, have recently led to the development of an ad hoc set of diagnostic criteria for patients with PPMS that incorporates the contribution from laboratory and MRI findings. In addition, several attempts have been or are being made to find an effective treatment for slowing the progression of PPMS. Disappointingly, but not unexpectedly, treatment able to modify favorably the course of other forms of MS has shown very little or no effect at all on the natural evolution of PPMS.

The issues of epidemiological and clinical characteristics as well as those relating to the pathology, immunology, experimental treatment and MR aspects of PPMS are all extensively and critically addressed in this book, which is based on the contributions from the most active researchers in the field of PPMS. The first chapter reports findings from the largest cohort of MS patients ever followed up for a period of more than 25 years and defines the epidemiological characteristics of PPMS, as well as the main prognostic factors for establishing a long-term clinical outcome. The second and the third chapters review the state of the art of the pathological and immunological aspects of PPMS and bring additional evidence to the notion that PPMS is part of the broad spectrum of MS rather than being a separate disease entity. In Chap. 4, the authors discuss the rationale and applications of neurophysiological techniques to the study of PPMS. The exquisite sensitivity of neurophysiological techniques for detecting and quantifying spinal cord damage indicates the importance of standardized neurophysiological protocols to increase diagnostic confidence and to monitor the evolution of patients with PPMS. In Chap. 5, the prevalence and features of cognitive impairment in PPMS is addressed. Again, as is seen in the other clinical phenotypes of the disease, cognitive impairment is present in PPMS, and an accurate assessment of it is a preliminary prerequisite for correct management of these patients and for achieving a better understanding of how structural damage, as quantified using MR technology, results in clinical deficits. Chap. 6 provides an extensive picture of the baseline clinical and MRI features of the largest clinical trial ever conducted in PPMS, the currently ongoing double-blind trial of glatiramer acetate. The analysis of this dataset has already provided and is likely to continue to provide important clues about the characteristics of the evolution of PPMS.

The remaining chapters of the book all deal with various MR features of PPMS. In Chap. 8, the conventional MRI findings are presented and their role in the diagnosis and monitoring of disease evolution, as well as reasons for the so-called "clinical/MRI paradox," are discussed in detail. Chapters 8 and 9 review the potential of quantitative nonconventional MR techniques in the study of structural damage in PPMS. Chap. 8 is an overview of the magnetization transfer and diffusion tensor MR studies conducted in patients with PPMS. It provides additional evidence on the role of microscopic brain damage and spinal cord pathology in contributing to the evolution of the disease. Chap. 9 is a meta-analysis and a review of all the available proton MR spectroscopy data in PPMS. It provides a strong background rationale for a future more extensive use of MR sectroscopy as a tool to assess in vivo the characteristics of axonal pathology in PPMS. The final chapter discusses how functional MRI holds substantial promise for improving our understanding of PPMS pathophysiology, by enabling us to investigate the presence and extent of adaptive cortical reorganization following tissue damage and, in consequence, to define the role of the failure of recovery mechanisms in causing the progressive accumulation of irreversible neurological disability.

This book is the result of an International workshop held in Milan on 26 May 2001, which was part of the Fifth Annual Advanced Course on the Use of Magnetic Resonance Techniques in Multiple Sclerosis. This workshop was an extensive and multidisciplinary discussion of the most recent findings in the field of PPMS research. Although, due to the nature of the workshop, more emphasis was given to new structural and functional MRI findings than to other aspects of the disease, we believe that the combination of epidemiological, pathological, immunological, neuropsychological, neurophysiological, and neuroimaging data presented in this book should provide the reader with a complete and up-to-date overview of what we have learned about PPMS in the past few years.

Chapter 1

Observations from the Natural History Cohort of London, Ontario

G. Rice, M. Kremenchutzky, D. Cottrell, J. Baskerville, G. Ebers

Introduction

Charcot recognized that a subset of patients with multiple sclerosis (MS) appeared to worsen in an insidiously progressive manner from the onset of the disease [1]. This clinically defined disease course has been called primary progressive multiple sclerosis (PPMS). There has been a tendency to consider this disease phenotype different from that of patients whose disease course is characterized by attacks, either relapsing-remitting MS (RRMS) or the late progressive phase of that condition, known as secondary progressive MS (SPMS) (Fig. 1). In contrast to RRMS, comparatively little information is available on the clinical and demographic features and the natural history of PPMS [2-5]. Prognostic variables have yet to be addressed specifically and the natural history has been less well charted.

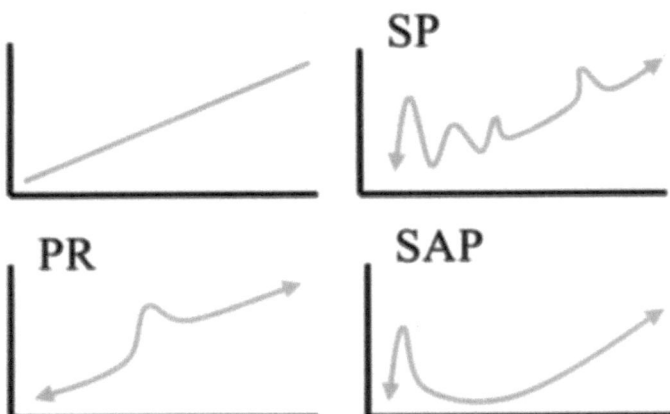

Fig. 1. Phenotypes of progressive MS. *PP*, primary progressive; *SP*, secondary progressive; *PR*, progressive-relapsing; *SAP*, single attack with later progression

Diagnostic Criteria

In the first studies which emanated from the London Natural History Study Group, patients were categorized as having RRMS, SPMS, or PPMS [6, 7]. The PPMS group originally included patients with purely progressive MS and some patients who experienced superimposed attacks, including both PPMS and progressive-relapsing MS (PRMS) according to a recent consensus [8]. We have studied the long-term natural history in this group and also in the subset of patients with superimposed relapses. The long-term prognosis does not appear to be different in those patients with progressive onset who have additional superimposed attacks [9].

Clinical Follow-Up in the London Multiple Sclerosis Clinic

The London Clinic has existed for almost 30 years. The characteristics of this clinic population have been outlined in previous publications [6, 7, 10]. The clinic population is concentrated here as a geographic base, with little referral bias and treatment. An inception cohort of 1099 patients, recruited between 1972 and 1984, has been followed on an annual basis. Most follow-up has been done directly. Follow-up data have been obtainable on more than 95% of the population. Of the original cohort of patients having or being reclassified as having PPMS, 96.6% are still considered to have MS.

The cohort of PPMS patients was constituted by 216 patients. All observations concerning baseline covariates in the original population have been validated in a more contemporary series of 165 PPMS patients who were identified between 1992 and 1997. The methodology and statistical approach have been well described elsewhere [6, 7, 10]. We have addressed these primary questions.

Are the Baseline Demographics and Clinical Features of PPMS Different From Those of the Other Phenotypes?

The mean age at onset of the PPMS patients was 38.5 years and the mean and median disease durations were 23.7 and 23.0 years, respectively – onset was approximately a decade later than in other forms of MS. Females still dominated this phenotype (ratio male:female 1:1.3), but less so than in the other phenotypes (ratio male:female 1:2). The ratio between males and females in PPMS fell with advancing age at onset, with the ratio again approaching 1:2 for later onset (Fig. 2).

The most common presenting symptom was motor deficit, seen in 109 (38.9%) patients, followed by sensory impairment in 91 (32.5%), cerebellar symptoms in 45 (16%), and brainstem difficulties in 15 (5.3%). Optic neuropathy was uncommon (4.3%). The median time from onset of symptoms to diagnosis was 8 years, although this has been reduced by half in the more recently studied cohort. Most patients (75%) had not been treated, and even the treatments which had been deployed are not considered to be effective today.

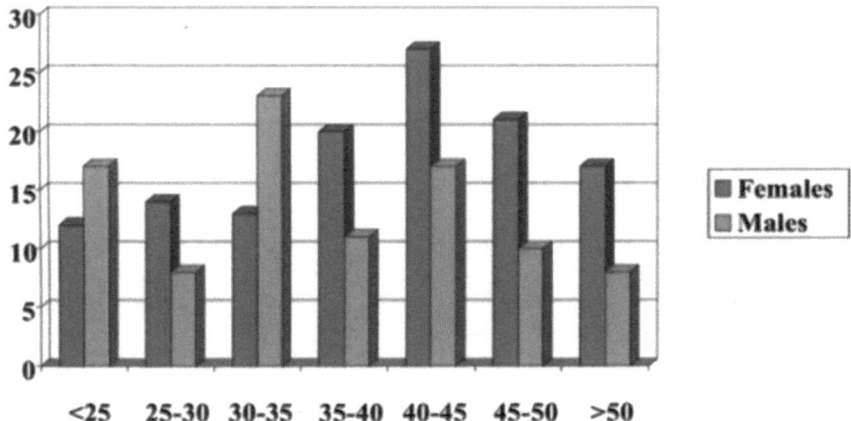

Fig. 2. Patient age at onset of PPMS

Are There Prognostic Variables at Baseline Which Anticipate a More Sinister Prognosis?

Two subpopulations of PPMS patients were identified as having a worse prognosis. This was particularly the case among those who had multiple systems involved at onset. If a patient had three or more systems involved at onset compared with one system, cane dependence (DSS 6) was reached sooner, by a median difference of 5 years, chair dependence (DSS 8) by 10 years, and death (DSS 10) by approximately 20 years. This observation was supported by data from the second series of PPMS patients.

Early accrual of a disability also anticipated further disease progression. If a patient reached mild disability (DSS 3) in less than 2 years, compared to more than 2 years (an interval which actually split the study population into halves), there was a reduction in time by around 5 years in the median time to chair confinement (DSS 8). This finding was consistent with previous observations [6, 7] which suggested that the time to DSS 3 in an unselected MS population affected long-term prognosis, and with data of Runmarker and Andersen [5], which suggested that in non-PPMS patients a low disability score after 5 years was a favorable prognostic indicator.

Is the Clinical Course of PPMS Different from That of the Other Phenotypes?

The probability of avoiding progression is shown for time to DSS landmark 6 (cane; Fig. 3), DSS 8 (chair; not shown), and DSS 10 (grave; not shown). The sur-

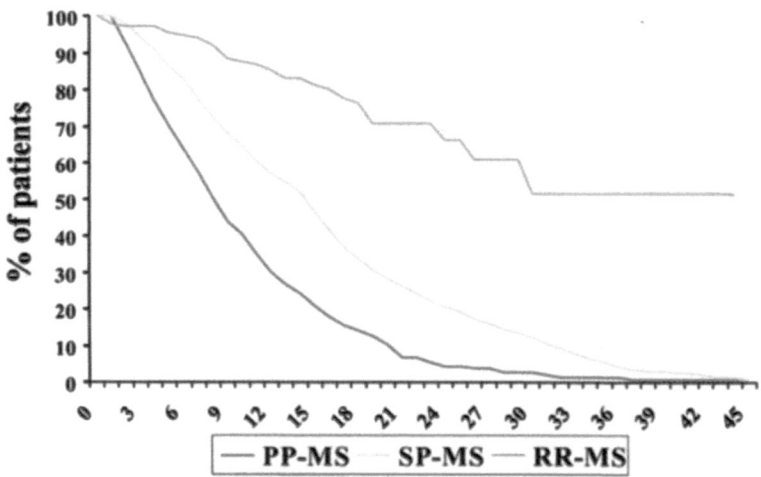

Fig. 3. Probability of avoiding DSS landmark 6 (one cane) with time after onset

vival curves are shown also for SPMS and RRMS. From the onset of the disease, the prognosis was clearly worse for patients with PPMS.

When the progression of the disease was plotted, after the onset of disease progression (generally at DSS 2-3), there was little difference among the PPMS patients, the SPMS patients, and a subset of SPMS patients who had experienced only a single attack before later disease progression (SAP-MS) (Fig. 4).

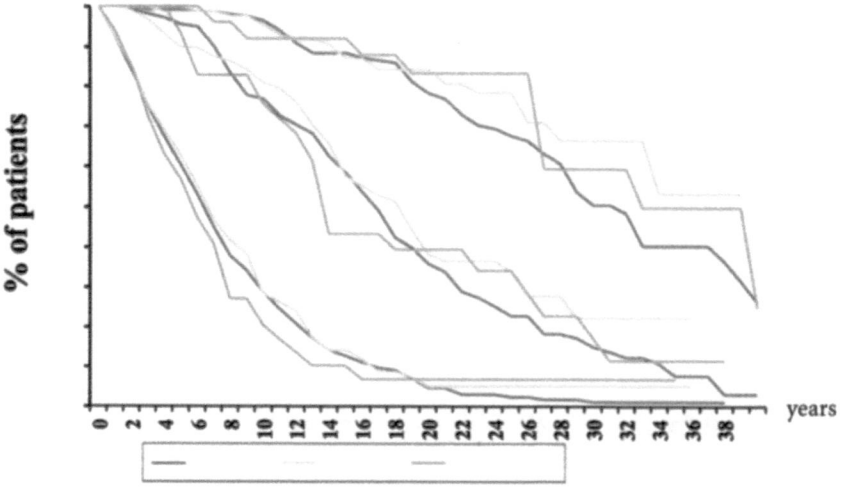

Fig. 4. Probability of avoiding DSS landmarks 6, 8, and 10 (cane, chair, death) with time in years after onset of disease progression

Is There a Difference Between PPMS and PRMS?

There did not appear to be a difference in the clinical course between MS patients whose progressive disease course was punctuated by attacks and those whose course was not. Survival curves of PP and PR subgroups were compared and were almost identical for the time from the onset of MS to DSS 8 ($p = 0.43$) or to death from MS (DSS 10) ($p = 0.62$). Closer scrutiny of the PR patients showed that some 50% "relapsed" within 10 years, 40% between 10 and 20 years, and 10% after 20 years (maximum 39 years). Most patients experienced good recovery from these attacks.

Are PPMS Patients Genetically Different?

This can be only partially answered by surveying recurrence rates for MS in patient families. Of the PPMS patients, 10.6% had a relative with MS, compared with 13.9% of the non-PPMS patients. This was not statistically significant ($p = 0.09$). We are in the process of studying the concordance of clinical phenotypes in MS sibling pairs and multiplex families. Some investigators have identified some immunogenetic differences between PPMS and RRMS patients [11]; further work in this area is needed.

Should We Subdivide MS?

It would be reasonable to ask whether the segregation of MS into distinct categories using phenotypic definitions is anything more than a descriptive exercise. Using the widely used definitions, there is considerable overlap among the clinical subgroups. Not all patients fit comfortably into the currently accepted definitions. It is possible that a phenotypic classification would divide a group of heterogeneous disorders artificially without imposing any greater order.

References

1. Charcot JM (1877) Disseminated sclerosis: its symptomatology. In: Charcot JM. Lectures on the diseases of the nervous system. London: New Sydenham Society, pp. 209-217
2. Confavreux C, Aimard G, Devic M (1980) Course and prognosis of multiple sclerosis assessed by the computerized data processing of 349 patients from the equalts. Brain 103:281-300
3. Poser S, Poser W, Schlaf G et al (1986) Prognostic indicators in multiple sclerosis. Acta Neurol Scand 74:387-392
4. Minderhoud JM, van der Hoeven JH, Prange AJ (1988) Course and prognosis of chronic progressive multiple sclerosis. Results of an epidemiological study. Acta Neurol Scand 78:10-15

5. Runmarker B, Andersen O (1993) Prognostic factors in a multiple sclerosis incidence cohort with twenty-five years of follow-up. Brain 116:117-134
6. Weinshenker BG, Bass B, Rice GP et al (1989) The natural history of multiple sclerosis: a geographically based study. 1. Clinical course and disability. Brain 112:133-146
7. Weinshenker BG, Bass B, Rice GP et al (1989) The natural history of multiple sclerosis: a geographically based study. 2. Predictive value of the early clinical course. Brain 112:1419-1428
8. Lublin FD, Reingold SC (1996) Defining the clinical course of multiple sclerosis: results of an international survey. Neurology 46:907-911
9. Kremenchutzky M, Cottrell D, Rice G et al (1999) The natural history of multiple sclerosis: a geographically based study. 7. Progressive-relapsing and relapsing-progressive multiple sclerosis: a re-evaluation. Brain 122:1941-1950
10. Weinshenker BG, Rice GP, Noseworthy JH et al (1991) The natural history of multiple sclerosis: a geographically based study. 3. Multivariate analysis of predictive factors and models of outcome. Brain 114: 1045-1056
11. Olerup O, Hillert J, Fredrikson S et al (1989) Primarily chronic progressive and relapsing/remitting multiple sclerosis: two immunogenetically distinct disease entities. Proc Natl Acad Sci USA 86:7113-7117

Chapter 2

Pathology

W. Brück

Introduction

Multiple sclerosis (MS) is a chronic inflammatory demyelinating disease of the central nervous system (CNS). The pathological hallmarks are the destruction of myelin, the death of oligodendrocytes, and the loss of axons [1, 2]. These changes occur against an inflammatory background which consists of inflammatory infiltrates composed of macrophages, microglia, and T and B cells, and is accompanied by an intense reaction of astrocytes leading to the typical glial scar formation of the chronic MS lesion. The lesions are scattered throughout the CNS, with a predilection for the optic nerves, brainstem, spinal cord, cerebellum, and periventricular white matter. Despite years of classical histopathological study and more recent intensive use of magnetic resonance technology, the MS lesion is incompletely understood [3]. How it is initiated, how it changes over time, and how it correlates with clinical symptoms or clinical course are all largely unknown. Therefore, it is essential that the evolution of the MS lesion is better understood and its clinical and paraclinical correlates defined.

Clinically, there is a broad spectrum of signs and symptoms that can occur in MS. The clinical course, the nature of symptoms, the chance of remission, and the response to therapy may be extremely variable between patients. Besides this clinical variability, substantial pathological heterogeneity has also been described, which most likely reflects different immunopathogenic disease mechanisms. The clinical heterogeneity already has, and the immunopathogenic heterogeneity certainly will have, important implications for further treatment efforts. From a clinical perspective, subgroups of MS patients may be defined on the basis of the time course of symptom development [4]. Most often, during the first years of the disease symptoms come and go, and this disease course has therefore been called "relapsing-remitting" (RRMS). In about 80% of patients, the illness begins in this way. Most patients who initially had a relapsing-remitting course move on into a secondary progressive (SPMS) stage after a number of years. Only 10%-20% of patients have continuously progressing symptoms from the beginning of their disease. This kind of disease course is called "primary progressive" (PPMS). In PPMS patients, the disease starts later in life, males are as frequently affected as females, the prognosis is worse, there may be more lesions in the spinal cord than in the brain, and the immunogenetic profile is different [5, 6].

From the pathological point of view, very few studies have focused on the question of whether a defined clinical subtype is also characterized by a specific pathology. This problem is mainly due to the fact that most pathological studies deal with chronic autopsy cases in which clinical documentation of the patients may be insufficient. Therefore, most studies do not separate the patients according to their clinical disease course, but only distinguish between acute and chronic MS. The other point is that lesions may go through different stages of activity in the course of their evolution and the definition of lesional activity in MS is not used uniformly in the literature [7]. Therefore, studies are often difficult to compare to each other. In the next section, the current knowledge of the pathological features of PPMS is summarized with special focus on inflammation, oligodendrocyte/myelin pathology, axonal destruction, and immunopathology of the MS lesion.

Inflammation

The inflammatory infiltrate of the MS lesion is composed of CD4+ and CD8+ T cells, B cells, plasma cells, hematogenous macrophages, and activated resident microglial cells [8]. The main portion of the infiltrate is formed by the macrophage/microglia population within the plaque, followed in number by T cells and plasma cells [9]. Only a few studies have examined whether the inflammatory components of the MS lesion are differently distributed in the different disease courses. A careful study revealed a significantly lower amount of inflammation in PPMS than in SPMS lesions [10]. This difference was detected in lesions of the cerebral hemispheres, the brainstem, and the spinal cord and may correlate with the lower frequency of gadolinium-enhancing lesions observed in PPMS. These data have been confirmed in our own clinical experience of MS (Fig. 1a). Various mechanisms may account for this difference, including a less severe or shorter-lived inflammation in PPMS. Apoptosis of lymphocytes appears to be a major mechanism for the resolution of inflammation in MS. This so-called programmed cell death is regulated by a panel of inhibitory or promoting proteins which include the bcl-2 protein, a major antiapoptotic molecule. This protein has been shown to be expressed by T lymphocytes in MS plaques, and patients with PPMS have a higher proportion of bcl-2-expressing T cells in their lesions [11]. This observation suggests impaired elimination of T cells from PPMS lesions. Thus, inflammation in PPMS may be less severe but persist for longer in the CNS than occurs with RRMS and SPMS lesions.

A recent investigation into the numbers of macrophages/microglia in the different disease courses confirmed the known data on lymphocytes in MS lesions, with the lowest numbers seen in PPMS (Fig. 1b). Macrophages are the main cells responsible for myelin uptake in the lesions. It is not clear whether macrophages of patients with PPMS are characterized by a different immunological activation pattern and, therefore, by a different capacity to remove myelin in the lesions. There are differences in adhesion molecule expression by leukocytes in the dif-

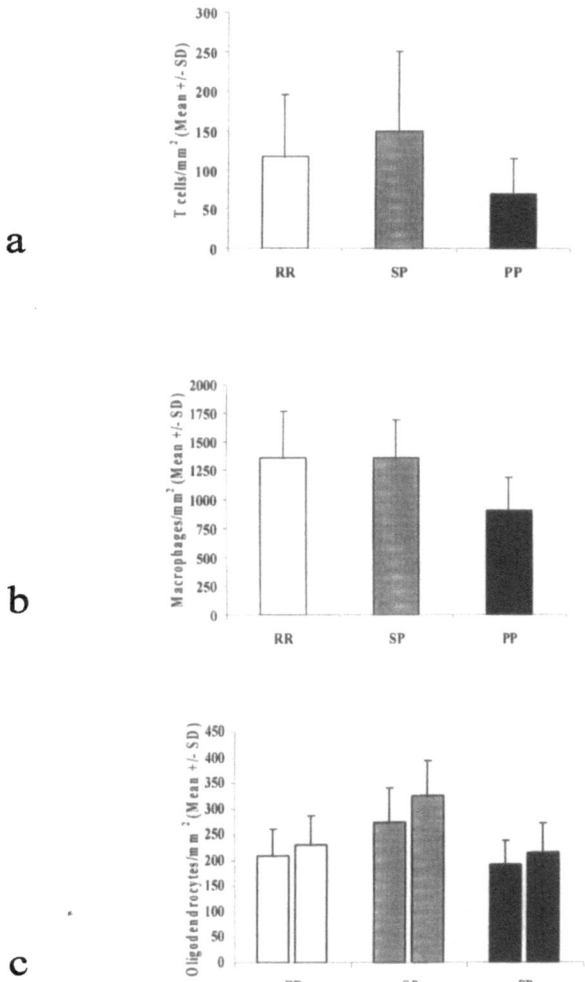

Fig. 1. Quantitative analysis of T cells (a), macrophages (b) and oligodendrocytes (c) in relapsing-remitting (*white*), secondary progressive (*gray*), and primary progressive MS (*black*). Oligodendrocyte numbers in c correspond to cells expressing myelin oligodendrocyte glycoprotein (*left hand columns*) or proteolipidprotein mRNA (*right hand columns*)

ferent disease courses [12], and urinary myelin basic protein-like material was found to be significantly lower in PPMS patients than in SPMS patients [13]. Whether these observations indicate a lower activation status of macrophages in PPMS remains to be established.

Oligodendrocyte/Myelin Pathology

After careful histopathological evaluation of biopsy and autopsy lesions of a large series of MS patients, two distinct patterns of myelin and oligodendrocyte pathology were distinguished [14]. The first showed reduction of oligodendrocytes in lesions with ongoing active demyelination and reappearance of oligodendrocytes after resolution of active demyelination, leading to remyelination in a substantial number of lesions. Most of these "new" oligodendrocytes may have emerged from the oligodendrocyte progenitor pool. The second pattern revealed severe destruction of oligodendrocytes without reappearance and remyelination. There were no major differences in the number of oligodendrocytes with respect to different disease courses. However, there was a trend towards lower oligodendrocyte numbers in PPMS and progressive-relapsing MS (PRMS) (Fig. 1c).

During the demyelinating process, oligodendrocytes are generally lost, especially in the chronic disease stages. Apoptosis is also involved in this process and, as mentioned above, the antiapoptotic protein bcl-2 is the main inhibitory molecule in the complex network of apoptosis. The expression of this protein in MS lesions was significantly associated with oligodendrocyte survival [15]. Looking at different disease courses, RRMS and SPMS patients had the highest numbers of bcl-2-expressing oligodendrocytes, compared to the few cases of PPMS examined in this study. This may, however, imply a higher vulnerability of oligodendrocytes in PPMS patients.

Immunopathology

Knowledge of the heterogeneity of oligodendrocyte/myelin pathology as described above suggested that the pathological events leading to myelin and/or oligodendrocyte injury in MS are variable and may be due to different immunological, toxic, or degenerative mechanisms. This hypothesis is supported by data from the animal model of MS, experimental autoimmune encephalomyelitis, and from in vitro studies, in which a large panel of different effectors was shown to damage oligodendrocytes and myelin. Therefore, a follow-up study of active demyelinating MS lesions aimed at identifying the presence of different pathways leading to myelin/oligodendrocyte damage was designed. After analysis of cellular inflammatory infiltrates and expression of inflammatory mediator molecules, four distinct immunopathogenetic subtypes were identified and conclusions about possible disease mechanisms were drawn [16, 17] as follows:

– Pattern I: T cell/macrophage-mediated demyelination
– Pattern II: antibody/complement-mediated demyelination
– Pattern III: oligodendrocyte dystrophy with myelin protein dysregulation and oligodendrocyte apoptosis
– Pattern IV: primary oligodendrocyte degeneration with features similar to those of viral infection or toxic oligodendrocyte damage, but not to those of autoimmunity.

An essential point is that there was heterogeneity between patients, but that only one distinct pattern was observed in multiple active demyelinating lesions in an individual patient at the time of tissue investigation. Whether these patterns change over time during the further evolution of the disease is not yet clear. Patterns I-III were distributed fairly homogenously among the different disease courses. In contrast, pattern IV was exclusively observed in three cases of PPMS. This may indicate that specific oligodendrocyte damage is present in at least a subgroup of PPMS. This might occur against a genetic background that favors metabolic disturbances or dysregulation of the oligodendrocyte cell cycle regulation in the context of an inflammatory process.

Axon Pathology

The pathology of axons in MS has recently gained a lot of attention, although it was mentioned even in the earliest descriptions of the disease [18]. Axonal pathology seems to play a major role in the development of clinical disability in MS patients [19]. Axonal density is reduced in most MS plaques and occurs in two phases. Acute axonal pathology may occur during active demyelination, and may already be apparent at the earliest stages of disease evolution, as described in several MS neuropathological studies. Ferguson et al. [20] examined MS lesions immunocytochemically for expression of amyloid precursor protein (APP), a marker of early axonal damage. They demonstrated extensive axonal damage throughout acute plaques and at the margins of active chronic plaques. Areas containing inflammation, demyelination, and macrophage infiltration were located close to one another, suggesting that axonal damage was closely associated with inflammation. A subsequent study by Trapp et al. [21] demonstrated abundant evidence of axonal transection in active MS lesions and suggested that this may be the pathological correlate of the irreversible neurological impairment seen in the disease [21]. The mechanisms leading to acute axonal damage are unknown. In a recent study [22], the extent of axonal injury correlated with the number of macrophages and CD8+ T cells in the lesions. It has also been suggested that antibodies to axonal proteins are involved in mediating axonal damage. Antiganglioside antibodies might participate in this process, and they were found in significantly higher number in PPMS than in SPMS or RRMS [23]. Bitsch et al. [22] also studied whether there are differences between the different disease groups and found significantly higher amounts of acutely damaged axons in SPMS than in PPMS lesions.

To summarize, at present there are few data available on the specific pathology of PPMS. These data indicate the existance of both a qualitative and a quantitative difference between the different disease courses. The qualitative difference is the occurrence of one immunopathological subtype of demyelination, namely primary oligodendrocyte degeneration, in a subgroup of PPMS patients. The quantitative one is less severe inflammation, more pronounced oligodendrocyte loss, and ongoing low-level axonal damage in PPMS.

References

1. Prineas JW (1985) The neuropathology of multiple sclerosis. In: Koetsier JC (ed) Demyelinating diseases. Elsevier Science, Amsterdam, pp 213-257
2. Lassmann H (1998) Pathology of multiple sclerosis. In: Compston A, Ebers G, Lassmann H et al (eds) McAlpine's multiple mclerosis. Churchill Livingstone, London, pp 323-358
3. Lucchinetti C, Brück W, Noseworthy JH (2001) Multiple sclerosis: recent developments in neuropathology, pathogenesis, magnetic resonance imaging and treatment. Curr Opin Neurol 14:259-269
4. Lublin FD, Reingold SC (1996) Defining the clinical course of multiple sclerosis: results of an international survey. Neurology 46:907-911
5. Thompson AJ, Montalban X, Barkhof F et al (2000) Diagnostic criteria for primary progressive multiple sclerosis: a position paper. Ann Neurol 47:831-835
6. Thompson AJ, Polman CH, Miller DH et al (1997) Primary progressive multiple sclerosis. Brain 120:1085-1096
7. Lassmann H, Raine CS, Antel J, Prineas JW (1998) Immunopathology of multiple sclerosis: report on an international meeting held at the Institute of Neurology of the University of Vienna. J Neuroimmunol 86:213-217
8. Traugott U, Reinherz EL, Raine CS (1983) Multiple sclerosis. Distribution of T cells, T cell subsets and Ia-positive macrophages in lesions of different ages. J Neuroimmunol 4:201-221
9. Brück W, Porada P, Poser S et al (1995) Monocyte/macrophage differentiation in early multiple sclerosis lesions. Ann Neurol 38:788-796
10. Revesz T, Kidd D, Thompson AJ, Barnard RO, McDonald WI (1994) A comparison of the pathology of primary and secondary progressive multiple sclerosis. Brain 117:759-765
11. Zettl UK, Kuhlmann T, Brück W (1998) Bcl-2 expressing T lymphocytes in multiple sclerosis lesions. Neuropathol Appl Neurobiol 24:202-208
12. Durán I, Martinez-Cáceres EM, Rio J et al (1999) Immunological profile of patients with primary progressive multiple sclerosis. Expression of adhesion molecules. Brain 122:2297-2307
13. Bashir K, Whitaker JN (1999) Clinical and laboratory features of primary progressive and secondary progressive MS. Neurology 53:765-771
14. Lucchinetti C, Brück W, Parisi J et al (1999) A quantitative analysis of oligodendrocytes in multiple sclerosis lesions. A study of 113 cases. Brain 122:2279-2295
15. Kuhlmann T, Lucchinetti C, Zettl UK et al (1999) Bcl-2-expressing oligodendrocytes in multiple sclerosis lesions. Glia 28:34-39
16. Lucchinetti C, Brück W, Parisi J et al (2000) Heterogeneity of multiple sclerosis lesions: implications for the pathogenesis of demyelination. Ann Neurol 47:707-717
17. Lassmann H, Brück W, Lucchinetti C (2001) Heterogeneity of multiple sclerosis pathogenesis: implications for diagnosis and therapy. Trends Mol Med 7:115-121
18. Kornek B, Lassmann H (1999) Axonal pathology in multiple sclerosis. A historical note. Brain Pathol 9:651-656
19. Trapp BD, Ransohoff R, Rudick R (1999) Axonal pathology in multiple sclerosis: relationship to neurologic disability. Curr Opin Neurol 12:295-302
20. Ferguson B, Matyszak MK, Esiri MM, Perry VH (1997) Axonal damage in acute multiple sclerosis lesions. Brain 120:393-399
21. Trapp BD, Peterson J, Ransohoff RM et al (1998) Axonal transection in the lesions of multiple sclerosis. N Engl J Med 338:278-285
22. Bitsch A, Schuchardt J, Bunkowski S et al (2000) Axonal injury in multiple sclerosis. Correlation with demyelination and inflammation. Brain 123:1174-1183
23. Sadatipour BT, Greer JM, Pender MP (1998) Increased circulating antiganglioside antibodies in primary and secondary progressive multiple sclerosis. Ann Neurol 44:980-983

Chapter 3

Immunology

X. Montalban

Introduction

Multiple sclerosis (MS) is a chronic inflammatory demyelinating disease of the central nervous system (CNS). Three major clinical courses have been identified in MS: relapsing-remitting MS (RRMS), characterized by exacerbations with subsequent total or partial remission of symptoms; secondary progressive MS (SPMS), in which progression follows an initial RRMS phase; and primary progressive MS (PPMS), a progressive form without relapses or remissions [1]. Although by definition PPMS is clinically different from the relapsing forms, in the past, the SPMS and PPMS forms were grouped together as "chronic progressive" (CPMS) MS. However, in the first magnetic resonance imaging (MRI) study in which PPMS was specifically investigated, it was shown that patients with PPMS, despite marked disability, had fewer and smaller gadolinium-enhancing cerebral MRI lesions than patients with SPMS [2, 3]. Furthermore, a more recent study of a large cohort of PPMS patients from six European centres has shown clear differences in MRI appearances between PPMS and SPMS [4]. Few papers have addressed the pathological differences between PPMS and the relapsing forms; inflammation, though less marked, is also obviously present in PPMS lesions [5]. Although a small number of patients with PPMS could have a distinct pathological pattern, the samples studied are small, and some cases of PPMS are indistinguishable from RR forms of MS [6]. While MS is generally associated with the haplotype A3-B7-DR2 (15)-DQw6, this occurs predominantly with the RR form of the disease. Although there is some evidence that PPMS may be associated with DR4, the relationship is still inconsistent.

The clinical, pathological, and radiological evidence suggests that PPMS may differ from the relapsing forms, which include RRMS and SPMS. Nevertheless, few studies have been devoted to investigating the specific immunological features that may be found in PPMS patients [7-16]. This is mainly due to the fact that in most published studies patients with CPMS have not been subdivided into PPMS and SPMS subgroups. These immunological markers would allow more specific targeting of immunotherapies.

It has been described that PPMS patients have oligoclonal bands in their cerebrospinal fluid (CSF) [7], increased levels of antiganglioside antibodies [8, 9], or soluble adhesion molecules [10-13] less frequently than the other clinical subgroups. In this chapter, some immunological studies recently performed will be reviewed.

Cytokines

Cytokines are soluble peptides that mediate intercellular communication. Evidence showing the importance of cytokines in the pathogenesis of MS is mounting. Classically, MS has been considered a CD4+ Th1-lymphocyte-mediated disease, producing proinflammatory cytokines such as IFN-γ, TNF-α, or TNF-β, which stimulate macrophages and can destroy or mediate injury of target cells. Furthermore, IFN-α and TNF-β can induce the expression of MHC-II and adhesion molecules, allowing T cells to interact with the endothelium at the blood-brain barrier (BBB). An increase in IFN-γ and TNF-α has been found in serum of MS patients prior to clinical relapses [17, 18], and in situ messenger RNA of these cytokines has been detected during the acute phase of the disease in the context of experimental autoimmune encephalomyelitis (EAE), an animal model of MS [19, 20]. It has also been reported that treatment of MS patients with recombinant IFN-γ induced exacerbations of the disease [21]. In the same manner, an increase of IL-12, the most potent inducer of IFN-γ, has been associated with disease activity in patients with progressive MS [22-24].

IL-1 and IL-6 have been shown to have costimulatory activity on T cell activation [25]. Recently, we demonstrated that IFNβ-1b treatment increases the percentage of IL-6-producing cells by the third month of therapy in RRMS patients. This increase was significant in patients who developed flu-like symptoms with fever during the first weeks of treatment, the symptoms becoming milder when treated with low-dose oral steroids [26]. Proinflammatory cytokines are regulated by inhibitory cytokines such as IL-4, TGF-β, or IL-10. In EAE, signs of disease were decreased or abrogated by treatment with these cytokines [27-31].

It is tempting to speculate that production and release of cytokines differ in the individual clinical forms. At least two research groups have presented data on cytokine production in the different clinical forms of MS. Killestein et al. [15] studied 72 patients with MS (24 RRMS, 26 SPMS, 22 PPMS) and observed that PPMS patients display a significant decrease in CD4+ T cells producing IL-2, IL-13, and TNF-α and a significant increase in CD [8] T cells producing IL-4 and IL-10. On the other hand, after a preliminary study where we observed increased production of IFN-γ by lymphocytes of relapsing forms but not of PPMS [14], we compared in a larger number of patients (24 PPMS, 20 RRMS, 21 SPMS) and 29 healthy controls the ability of peripheral blood mononuclear cells (PBMC) to produce cytokines in response to mitogenic stimulation [16]. The capability of PBMC to produce IFN-γ and TNF-α (in the T cell subpopulation) and IL-6, IL-10, and IL-12 (in the monocyte/macrophage population) was tested by flow cytometry. No significant differences were observed either in percentage or in mean fluorescence intensity between the MS group and the healthy controls in any of the cytokines studied. We did not find significant differences in the percentage of cytokine-producing cells between PPMS and healthy controls; although we observed a slight increase in the percentage of IL-6-producing cells in RRMS and SPMS patients in relation to PPMS and healthy controls, it did not reach statistical significance. In the same way, when analyzing the mean fluorescence intensity per cell, we did not observe statistically significant differences between groups in relation to IFN-γ, TNF-α, IL-6, IL-10, or IL-12 production. In this context, Rovaris et al. [32], analyzing soluble cytokines (IL-1, IL-6, TNF-α) by ELISA, did not find any differences in serum or CSF cytokine levels among RRMS, SPMS, and PPMS.

Adhesion Molecules

Adhesion molecules play an important role in the migration of peripheral leukocytes into the CNS [33]. In EAE, adhesion molecules have been extensively shown to play a central role in the pathogenesis of the disease [34-36] and that, at the same time, antibodies against different adhesion molecules inhibit EAE [37-42]. Based on their structure, adhesion molecules are classified into selectins, integrins, and members of the immunoglobulin (Ig) superfamily. Selectins are involved in the initial localization of leukocytes to inflammatory sites. Integrins and members of the Ig superfamily mediate strong adhesion and migration of leukocytes across the vascular endothelium [43].

Although a major role for adhesion molecules has been presumed in MS, where the ability of leukocytes to cross the BBB seems to be an early feature of enhancing lesions, most authors have analyzed individual adhesion molecules in specific subgroups of patients [44-48]. In relation to soluble forms in MS patients, several groups have reported elevated levels of soluble ICAM-1 (intercellular adhesion molecule-1, CD54), soluble L-selectin (CD62L), soluble VCAM-1 (vascular cell adhesion molecule, CD106), or soluble ICAM-3 (intercellular adhesion molecule-3, CD50) [10, 49-53]. Most of these studies subdivide MS patients into those with RRMS and those with CPMS. Just a few authors attempted an analysis of the three clinical forms (RRMS, SPMS, and PPMS) separately [11, 12, 54]. Giovannoni et al. found increased serum levels of soluble ICAM-1 in RRMS and SPMS, and insignificant levels in PPMS [10]. McDonnell et al. found no differences in the ICAM-1 and L-selectin indices among the different groups of patients [54]. In a later study, however, the same authors found increased levels of soluble ICAM-1 in PPMS in comparison to the other clinical forms of MS, and increased levels of L-selectin in RRMS [12]. We compared membrane expression of adhesion molecules ICAM-1 (CD54), LFA-1α (CD11a), VLA-4 [$α_4/β_1$ integrin (CD49d/CD29)], L-selectin (CD62L), and ICAM-3 (CD50) in peripheral blood and serum-soluble forms ICAM-1, L-selectin, VCAM-1, and ICAM-3 in 89 patients (39 PPMS, 25 SPMS, 25 RRMS) and 38 healthy controls. We found a significant decrease in leukocyte surface expression in most of the adhesion molecules tested and an increase in soluble ICAM-1 and L-selectin levels in SPMS and RRMS compared to PPMS, which was similar to controls [13]. These results support the supposition that, as suspected from MRI findings, migration of autoreactive leukocytes through the BBB would be crucial to the pathogenesis of SPMS and RRMS, whereas other mechanisms leading to progressive axonal damage would account for the primary progressive form of the disease.

Chemokines

Chemokines constitute a large family of small chemoattractant cytokines that share important structural features and the ability to attract leukocytes. The regulated interactions of chemokines with their respective cell surface receptors mediate the recruitment of specific leukocyte subpopulations to sites of inflammation [55]. A number of studies have demonstrated the expression of several chemokines such as MCP-1, MCP-2, MCP-3, MIP-1β, MIP-1α, RANTES, Mig, and IP-10 as well as chemokine receptors in lesions at different stages of MS [56-58] and there are several reports on the association between an increase in chemokine/chemokine receptor expression in the CNS of MS patients and neurological dysfunction. Sorensen et al. [62], who analyzed patients with active disease, found consistent alterations of two ligand-receptor systems: IP-10/Mig-CXCR3 and RANTES-CCR5. Also, in patients during the course of a clinical relapse, higher CSF levels of MIP-α have been reported in comparison to patients with noninflammatory neurological diseases [60]. Increased numbers of CCR5+ cells in MS patients during a relapse have also been described [61]. These findings have important implications for our understanding of the mechanisms underlying aberrant T cell traffic during relapses in MS. There are no studies analyzing chemokine/chemokine receptor expression specifically in RRMS, SPMS, and PPMS. Only Balashov et al. [62] showed an increase in CXCR3+ and CCR5+ cells in the peripheral blood together with an increase of MIP-1α and IP-10 in the CSF of patients with the CP forms of the disease. We have analyzed the membrane expression of a group of CC and CXC chemokine receptors (CCR1, CCR5, CXCR3, CXCR4) in peripheral blood of 68 MS patients (25 PPMS, 23 SMPS, 20 RRMS) and 26 healthy controls. In a subgroup of patients, the CSF levels of IP-10 and RANTES chemokines were also analyzed. A significant increase of surface expression of CCR5 in CD4+, CD8+, CD19+, and CD14+ cells as well as an increased percentage of CXCR3 and CXCR4 in CD14+ cells were observed in MS patients compared to the control group. CSF levels of IP-10 were also significantly increased in MS patients compared to controls. These results support the supposition that chemokines and their receptors are involved in the pathogenesis of MS. However, a characteristic pattern of chemokine/chemokine receptor expression for the different clinical forms of the disease was not observed.

Conclusions

Tempting though it is to speculate that PPMS and relapsing forms of MS differ in their immunological patterns, the data are still not fully convincing and the search for immunological and biological markers of the various forms of MS needs to continue.

References

1. Lublin FD, Reingold SC (1996) Defining the clinical course of multiple sclerosis: results of an international survey. Neurology 46:907-910
2. Thompson AJ, Miller DH, MacManus DG, McDonald WI (1990) Patterns of disease activity in multiple sclerosis: a clinical and magnetic resonance imaging study. Br Med J 300:631-634
3. Thompson AJ, Polman CH, Miller DH et al (1997) Primary progressive multiple sclerosis. Brain 120:1085-1096
4. Stevenson VL, Miller DH, Rovaris M et al (1999) Primary progressive and transitional progressive multiple sclerosis: a clinical and MRI cross sectional study. Neurology 52:839-845
5. Revesz T, Kidd D, Thompson AJ et al (1994) A comparison of the pathology of primary and secondary progressive multiple sclerosis. Brain 117:759-765
6. Lucchinetti C, Bruck W, Parisi J et al (2000). Heterogeneity of multiple sclerosis lesions: implications for the pathogenesis of demyelination. Ann Neurol 47:707-717
7. Pirttila T, Nurmikko T (1995) CSF oligoclonal bands, MRI, and the diagnosis of multiple sclerosis. Acta Neurol Scand 92:468-71
8. Acarín N, Rio J, Fernandez AL et al (1996) Different antiganglioside antibody pattern between relapsing-remitting and progressive MS. Acta Neurol Scand 93:99-103
9. Sadatipour BT, Greer JM, Pender MP (1998) Increased circulating antiganglioside antibodies in primary and secondary progressive multiple sclerosis. Ann Neurol 44:980-983
10. Giovannoni G, Lai M, Thorpe J et al (1997) Longitudinal study of soluble adhesion molecules in multiple sclerosis: correlation with gadolinium enhanced magnetic resonance imaging. Neurology 48:1557-1565
11. Giovannoni G, Thorpe JW, Kidd D et al (1996) Soluble E-selectin in multiple sclerosis: raised concentrations in patients with primary progressive disease. J Neurol Neurosurg Psychiatry 60:20-26
12. McDonnell GV, McMillan SA, Douglas JP et al (1999) Serum soluble adhesion molecules in multiple sclerosis: raised sVCAM-1, sICAM-1 and sE-selectin in primary progressive disease. J Neurol 246:87-92
13. Durán I, Martinez-Caceres EM, Rio J et al (1999) Immunological profile of patients with primary progressive multiple sclerosis. Expression of adhesion molecules. Brain 122:2297-2307
14. Durán I, Martínez-Cáceres E, Barberà N et al (1998) Immunological profile of primary progressive multiple sclerosis. Mult Scler 4:348
15. Killestein J, Den Drijver BF, Van der Graaff WL et al (2001) Intracellular cytokine profile in T-cells subsets of multiple sclerosis patients: different fetures in primary progressive disease. Mult Scler 7:145-150
16. Durán I, Martinez-Caceres EM, Brieva L et al (2001) Similar pro- and anti-inflammatory cytokine production in the different clinical forms of multiple sclerosis. Mult Scler 7:151-156
17. Beck J, Rondot P, Catinot L et al (1988) Increased production of interferon gamma and tumor necrosis factor precedes clinical manifestations in multiple sclerosis: do cytokines trigger off exacerbations? Acta Neurol Scand 78:318-323
18. Chofflon M, Juillard C, Juillard P et al (1992) Tumor necrosis factor a production as a possible predictor of relapse in patients with multiple sclerosis. Eur Cytokine Netw 3:523-531
19. Issazadeh S, Ljungdahl A, Hojeberg B et al (1995) Cytokine production in the central nervous system of Lewis rats with experimental autoimmune encephalomyelitis: dynamics of mRNA expression for interleukin-10, interleukin-12, cytolysin, tumor necrosis factor alpha and tumor necrosis factor beta. J Neuroimmunol 61:205-212

20. Issazadeh S, Lorentzen JC, Mustafa MI et al (1996) Cytokines in relapsing experimental autoimmune encephalomyelitis in DA rats: persistent mRNA expression of proinflammatory cytokines and absent expression of interleukin-10 and transforming growth factor-beta. J Neuroimmunol 69:103-115

21. Panitch HS, Hirsch RL, Haley AS, Johnson KP (1987) Exacerbations of multiple sclerosis in patients treated with gamma-interferon. Lancet 1:893-896

22. Trinchieri G (1995) Interleukin 12: a proinflammatory cytokine with immunoregulatory functions that bridge innate resistance and antigen-specific adaptive immunity. Annu Rev Immunol 13:251-276

23. Correale J, McMillan M, Li S et al (1997) Antigen presentation by autoreactive proteolipid protein peptide-specific T cell clones from chronic progressive multiple sclerosis patients: roles of co-stimulatory B7 molecules and IL-12. J Neuroimmunol 72:27-43

24. Comabella M, Balashov K, Issazadeh S et al (1998) Elevated interleukin-12 in progressive multiple sclerosis correlates with disease activity and is normalized by pulse cyclophosphamide therapy. J Clin Invest 102:671-678

25. Houssiau FA, Coulie PG, Van Snick J (1989) Distinct roles of IL-1 and IL-6 human T cell activation. J Immunol 143:2520-2524

26. Martínez-Cáceres EM, Rio J, Barrau M et al (1998) Amelioration of flu-like symptoms at the onset of IFNβ-1b therapy in multiple sclerosis by low oral steroid use is related to a decrease in IL-6 induction. Ann Neurol 44:682-685

27. Cash E, Minty A, Ferrara P et al (1994) Macrophage-inactivation IL-13 suppresses experimental autoimmune encephalomyelitis in rats. J Immunol 153:4258-4267

28. Racke MK, Burnett D, Pak SH et al (1995) Retinoid treatment of experimental allergic encephalomyelitis. IL-4 production correlates with improved disease course. J Immunol 154:450-458

29. Racke MK, Sriram S, Carlino J et al (1993) Long-term treatment of chronic relapsing experimental allergic encephalomyelitis by transforming growth factor-beta2. J Neuroimmunol 46:175-183

30. Racke MK, Dhib-Jalbut S, Cannella B et al (1991) Prevention and treatment of chronic relapsing experimental allergic encephalomyelitis by transforming growth factor-beta1. J Immunol 146:3012-3017

31. Rott O, Fleischer B, Cash E (1994) Interleukin-10 prevents experimental allergic encephalomyelitis in rats. Eur J Immunol 24:1434-1440

32. Rovaris M, Barnes D, Woodrofe N et al (1996) Patterns of disease activity in MS patients: a study with quantitative gadolinium-enhanced brain MRI and cytokine measurement in different clinical subgroups. J Neurol 247:536-542

33. Springer TA (1994) Traffic signals for lymphocyte recirculation and leukocyte emigration: the multistep paradigm. Cell 76:301-314

34. Kuchroo VK, Martin CA, Greer JM et al (1993) Cytokines and adhesion molecules contribute to the ability of myelin proteolipid protein-specific T cell clones to mediate experimental allergic encephalomyelitis. J Immunol 151:4371-4382

35. Anderson JA, Lentsch AB, Hadjiminas DJ et al (1996) The role of cytokines, adhesion molecules, and chemokines in interleukin-2-induced lymphocytic infiltration in C57BL/6 Mice. J Clin Invest 97:1952-1959

36. Previtali SC, Archelos JJ, Hartung HP (1997) Modulation of the expression of integrins on glial cells during experimental autoimmune encephalomyelitis. A central role for TNF-alpha. Am J Pathol 151:1425-1435

37. Yednock TA, Cannon C, Fritz LC et al (1992) Prevention of experimental autoimmune encephalomyelitis by antibodies against alpha 4 beta 1 integrin. Nature 356:63-66

38. Dopp JM, Breneman SM, Olschowka JA (1994) Expression of ICAM-1, VCAM-1, L-selectin, and leukosialin in the mouse central nervous system during the induction and remission stages of experimental allergic encephalomyelitis. J Neuroimmunol 54:129-144

39. Steffen BJ, Butcher EC, Engelhardt B (1994) Evidence for involvement of ICAM-1 and

VCAM-1 in lymphocyte interaction with endothelium in experimental autoimmune encephalomyelitis in the central nervous system in the SJL/J mouse. Am J Pathol 145:189-201

40. Gordon EJ, Myers KJ, Dougherty JP et al (1995) Both anti-CD11a (LFA-1) and anti-CD11b (MAC-1) therapy delay the onset and diminish the severity of experimental autoimmune encephalomyelitis. J Neuroimmunol 62:153-160

41. Kobayashi Y, Kawai K, Honda H et al (1995) Antibodies against leukocyte function-associated antigen-1 and against intercellular adhesion molecule-1 together suppress the progression of experimental allergic encephalomyelitis. Cell Immunol 164:295-305

42. Soilu-Hanninen M, Roytta M, Salmi A, Salonen R (1997) Therapy with antibody against leukocyte integrin VLA-4 (CD49d) is effective and safe in virus-facilitated experimental allergic encephalomyelitis. J Neuroimmunol 72:95-105

43. Hohlfeld R (1997) Biotechnological agents for the immunotherapy of multiple sclerosis. Principle, problems and perspectives. Brain 120:865-916

44. Porrini AM, Gambi D, Malatesta G (1992) Memory and naive CD4+ lymphocytes in multiple sclerosis. J Neurol 239:437-440

45. Svenningsson A, Hansson GK, Andersen O et al (1993) Adhesion molecule expression on cerebrospinal fluid T lymphocytes: evidence for common recruitment mechanisms in multiple sclerosis, aseptic meningitis, and normal controls. Ann Neurol 34:155-161

46. Salmaggi A, Dufour A, Eoli M et al (1996) Low serum interleukin-10 levels in multiple sclerosis: further evidence for decreased systemic immunosupression? J Neurol 243:13-17

47. Stüber A, Martin R, Stone LA et al (1996) Expression pattern of activation and adhesion molecules on peripheral blood CD4+ T-lymphocytes in relapsing-remitting multiple sclerosis patients: a serial analysis. J Neuroimmunol 66:147-151

48. Lou J, Chofflon M, Juillard C et al (1997) Brain microvascular endothelial cells and leukocytes derived from patients with multiple sclerosis exhibit increased adhesion capacity. NeuroReport 8:629-633

49. Dore-Duffy P, Newman W, Balabanov R et al (1995) Circulating, soluble adhesion proteins in cerebrospinal fluid and serum of patients with multiple sclerosis: correlation with clinical activity. Ann Neurol 37:55-62

50. Hartung HP, Reiners K, Archelos JJ et al (1995) Circulating adhesion molecules and tumor necrosis factor receptor in multiple sclerosis: correlation with magnetic resonance imaging. Ann Neurol 38:186-193

51. Martin S, Rieckmann P, Melchers I et al (1995) Circulating forms of ICAM-3 (cICAM-3). Elevated levels in autoimmune diseases and lack of association with cICAM-1. J Immunol 154:1951-1955

52. Matsuda M, Tsukada N, Miyagi K, Yanagisawa N (1995) Increased levels of soluble vascular cell adhesion molecule-1 (VCAM-1) in the cerebrospinal fluid and sera of patients with multiple sclerosis and human T lymphotropic virus type-1 associated myelopathy. J Neuroimmunol 59:35-40

53. Franciotta D, Piccolo G, Zardini E et al (1997) Soluble CD8 and ICAM-1 in serum and CSF of MS patients treated with 6-methylprednisolone. Acta Neurol Scand 95:275-279

54. McDonnell GV, McMillan SA, Douglas JP et al (1998) Raised CSF levels of soluble ·adhesion molecules across the clinical spectrum of multiple sclerosis. J Neuroimmunol 85:186-192

55. Baggiolini M (1998) Chemokines and leukocyte traffic. Nature 392:565-568

56. McManus C, Berman JW, Brett FM et al (1998) MCP-1, MCP-2 and MCP-3 expression in multiple sclerosis lesions: an immunohistochemical and in situ hybridization study. J Neuroimmunol 86:20-29

57. Simpson JE, Newcombe J, Cuzner ML, Woodroofe MN (1998) Expression of monocyte chemoattractant protein-1 and other b-chemokines by resident glia and inflammatory cells in multiple sclerosis lesions. J Neuroimmunol 84:238-244

58. Simpson JE, Newcombe J, Cuzner ML, Woodroofe MN (2000) Expression of the inter-

feron-gamma-inducible chemokines IP-10 and Mig and their receptor, CXCR3, in multiple sclerosis lesions. Neuropathol Appl Neurobiol 26:133-142

59. Sorensen TL, Tani M, Jensen J et al (1999) Expression of specific chemokines and chemokine receptors in the central nervous system of multiple sclerosis patients. J Clin Invest 103:807-815

60. Miyagishi R, Kikuchi S, Fukazawa T, Tashiro K (1995) Macrophage inflammatory protein-1 alpha in the cerebrospinal fluid of patients with multiple sclerosis and other inflammatory neurological diseases. J Neurol Sci 129:223-227

61. Strunk T, Bubel S, Mascher B et al (2000) Increased numbers of CCR5+ interferon-gamma and tumor-necrosis factor-alpha secreting T lymphocytes in multiple sclerosis patients. Ann Neurol 47:269-273

62. Balashov KE, Rottman JB, Weiner HL, Hancock WW (1999) CCR5(+) and CXCR3(+) T cells are increased in multiple sclerosis and their ligands MIP-1alpha and IP-10 are expressed in demyelinating brain lesions. Proc Natl Acad Sci USA 96:6873-6878

Chapter 4

Neurophysiology

L. Leocani, G. Comi

Introduction

Neurophysiological methods, particularly evoked potentials (EPs), are widely employed in the functional assessment of multiple sclerosis (MS), since they provide a reliable, even though indirect, measure of the extent of demyelination or axonal loss in a given pathway. For this reason, they are used to define the involvement of sensory and motor pathways in the presence of vague disturbances, and to detect clinically silent lesions. The latter application of EPs has become greatly reduced since the development of magnetic resonance imaging (MRI) technology, which has a much higher sensitivity in detecting subclinical lesions. Nevertheless, the information provided by EPs is different from that provided by structural MRI techniques, since EPs are more strictly related to function. Disease severity assessed clinically well correlates with the extent of neurophysiological abnormalities [1, 2]. Neurophysiological studies specifically aimed at characterizing the primary progressive (PP) form of MS, particularly with respect to secondary progressive MS (SPMS), are lacking. In this chapter, we discuss the rationale and applications of neurophysiological methods to the study of PPMS.

Evoked Potentials

The pathological substrates of EP abnormalities in MS are demyelination and axonal loss [3-5]. In myelinated fibres, saltatory conduction of action potentials is determined by clustering of voltage-sensitive sodium channels within axon membranes at nodes of Ranvier and, to a much lesser extent, beneath the myelin sheaths [6]. Demyelination may produce conduction block [7-9], which is also caused by soluble mediators of inflammation [10, 11]. In areas with partial demyelination, slowing of conduction velocity and a prolonged refractory period with failure in transmitting high-frequency impulses [12] may occur. As a result, EP abnormalities can consist of delayed latency, morphological abnormalities, wave cancellation, amplitude reduction, and increased refractory period [13, 14]. Axonal loss, which is also an important feature of MS, especially of the progressive phases [15], also contributes to EP abnormalities [16]. Even though EP abnormalities may reveal subclinical lesions [14,17,18], their value in the diagnosis of definite MS still needs to be clarified [17], since it is much lower than that of MRI

[14]. More promising is the utilization of EPs in the assessment of disease severity. In a study of 40 patients with relapsing remitting (RR) MS and 13 with SPMS [19], spinal motor conduction time and the frequency of abnormalities of multimodal EPs were significantly longer in the SPMS patients than in controls and RRMS patients. Spinal motor conduction times also correlated directly with Expanded Disability Status Scale (EDSS) scores and pyramidal functional system scores, while brain lesion load did not correlate with disability scores in SPMS. The authors of the study suggested that disability in SPMS patients is mainly due to progressive involvement of the corticospinal tract within the spinal cord. Filippi et al. [2] compared brain MRI and multimodal EPs in patients with benign MS and SPMS; EP abnormalities were significantly more frequent and more severe in the latter group, in accordance with their greater disability. Similarly, Kira et al. [20] found a significantly higher frequency of abnormal records in visual, brainstem auditory, and somatosensory EPs in PPMS than in RRMS. Moreover, clinically unexpected abnormalities were significantly more common in PPMS than in RRMS for all the EP modalities. To correlate clinical and EP findings, conventional scores might provide some advantage over parametric values such as latency and amplitude, since the latter may be more influenced by test-retest variability [21] and do not allow consideration of absent components. Conventional scores have been used in a preliminary study [22] evaluating the correlation between multimodal EPs, brain MRI, and clinical involvement in 13 PPMS and 27 SPMS patients. For the analysis of EP abnormalities, each examination was scored according to the following criteria: normal = 0; increased latency of one or more main components = 1; absence of one or more main components = 2. Brain MRI abnormalities were scored according to the method proposed by Ormerod et al. [23]. As shown in Table 1, motor, lower limb somatosensory, and visual EPs were found to be the most frequently abnormal in both progressive MS groups. This distribution of abnormalities agrees with the results of a larger study based on 83 PPMS patients [24].

In our study [22], no significant difference was found between PPMS and SPMS

Table 1. Frequency of evoked potential abnormalities (%) in 40 patients with PPMS and SPMS. (Modified from [22])

	Total	PPMS	SPMS	p
VEP	87	84	89	n.s.
BAEP	50	38	53	n.s.
SEP upper limb	67	61	70	n.s.
SEP lower limb	92	84	96	n.s.
MEP	100	100	100	n.s.

VEP, visual evoked potentials; BAEP, brainstem auditory evoked potentials; SEP, sensory evoked potentials; MEP, motor evoked potentials

in terms of frequency and severity of abnormalities, even though brain MRI lesion load was significantly higher in the SPMS group. A significant correlation was found between visual, auditory, and motor EPs and the corresponding functional systems, quantified using the EDSS [25]. The lack of significant correlation between somatosensory EPs and the functional sensory system might be related to the fact that functional sensory score not only evaluates deep sensation (the one mainly assessed by the somatosensory EP) but also skin sensation, particularly in the case of sensory deficits corresponding to a score higher than 1. Clinical disability, measured using the EDSS [25], was correlated with motor and lower limb somatosensory EPs. No significant correlation was found between brainstem MRI lesion load and brainstem auditory EPs (BAEPs) or between retrochiasmatic lesions and visual EPs (VEPs). Only a significance trend was found for the correlation of brain MRI total lesion load with a global EP score. Finally, no correlation was found between brain MRI total lesion load and EDSS.

These results may allow the elaboration of some general considerations. First, in this study a moderate correlation was found between the severity of disability and global EP abnormalities or motor and somatosensory EP results. This is not surprising, since EDSS score is driven by the motor functional system, particularly for scores between 4 and 8. This suggests that it is advisable to consider, for correlation with disability, the combined results of all EPs using a global score, since EDSS includes all functional systems. Second, in our patient group the EP results correlated more significantly with clinical findings than did brain conventional MRI. Several reasons may be considered to explain this finding, including the lack of MRI examination of the spinal cord, which is very important in determining disability. In addition, conventional MRI lacks pathological specificity to the different pathological processes in MS (edema, demyelination, gliosis, axonal loss) which can determine different functional outcomes. Again, the correlation between EP parameters and clinical findings confirms the usefulness of EPs in the functional assessment of MS patients. As a consequence, the similarity of EP findings in the PPMS and SPMS patients suggests that the sensory and motor pathways assessed by EPs in the spinal cord, brainstem, and optic nerve were similarly involved in these two groups.

EPs could be useful not only in the assessment of severity of progressive MS, but also to monitor disease evolution. Sater et al. [26] performed a longitudinal study (mean follow-up 1.5 years) of BAEPs and VEPs in a group of 11 chronic progressive MS patients. P100 latency significantly increased, while the BAEP I-V interpeak latency, T2-weighted MRI lesion load, and EDSS score did not. These data suggest that VEPs may be more sensitive than clinical and conventional brain MRI measures in the detection of disease evolution in the progressive phases, although they need to be validated with a larger group sample. A conventional nonparametric score, the Evoked Potentials Abnormality Score (EPAS), has been used together with conventional brain MRI and EDSS to evaluate longitudinal changes in a 2-year follow-up study of 50 MS patients [27]. While MRI correlated significantly with EDSS only at the cross-sectional evaluation at year 1, the EPAS correlated significantly with EDSS and MRI at all the cross-sectional evaluations and longitudinally only with EDSS changes. Kidd et al. [28] evaluated longitudinally central motor conduction time and brain and cervical MRI by means of transcranial magnetic stimulation in a group of 10 PPMS and 10 SPMS patients. Cord atrophy was present in five PPMS and three SPMS patients. While SPMS patients had a higher brain MRI lesion load than PPMS patients, no significant group difference was present for cervical cord MRI lesion load, central motor conduction time, and disability. Central motor conduction time was weakly but significantly correlated with EDSS but not with the pyramidal functional system. Correlation with cervical cord lesions was present for the upper limb only. As the authors pointed out, the significance of correlation may have been reduced by the exclusion of four patients with absent motor EPs of the lower limbs. After 1 year, seven SPMS and eight PPMS patients had worsened. The increase in central motor conduction time did not correlate significantly with changes in cord lesions or area, but was present only in the four patients with an increased number of cord lesions. Future larger longitudinal clinical/EP correlation studies should be able to define the usefulness of EPs in the monitoring of progressive MS.

Other Neurophysiological Methods

Despite similar clinical and neurophysiological involvement of brainstem and optic and spinal sensory and motor pathways in PPMS and SPMS patients, several MRI studies have suggested that the brain is more severely involved in SPMS than in PPMS patients [29-32]. Standard EPs evaluate the main sensory and motor projection pathways, but do not provide information about the associative and commissural pathways, which constitute the great majority of the brain white matter, and the involvement of which is considered to be the major determinant of the cognitive impairment in MS. Cognitive function is impaired in about 50% of MS patients [33, 34]. The pattern of mental dysfunction is typical of subcortical dementia [35, 36], and it is explained by the disconnection of large proportions of cortical associative areas, occurring as a consequence of subcortical demyelination and axonal degeneration [36-38]. The importance of lesions immediately underlying cortex, with respect to other lesion locations, has also been considered [39, 40]. Cognitive impairment is less frequent in PPMS patients than in SPMS patients [32, 41], probably because of the lower brain lesion burden. Moreover, when PPMS and SPMS patients have similar disability and MRI lesion burden, as is the case among the patients studied by Foong et al. [42], the frequency and severity of cognitive disturbances do not significantly differ between the two MS phenotypes, confirming the role of cortical deafferentation in MS dementia.

The electroencephalogram (EEG), which is the expression of multiple neuronal network interactions affected by white matter damage, may be used as an indicator of the global status of such interactions [43]. Spectral analysis of the EEG revealed abnormalities in 40%-79% of MS patients [44, 45], mainly an increase of slow frequency and decrease of α band. In progressive MS patients, these abnormalities have been found by Leocani et al. [46] to be related to cognitive dysfunction. In that study, EEG spectral power and coherence were examined in a group of 28 progressive MS patients (16 PPMS, 12 SPMS) with or without cognitive impairment assessed by a battery of neuropsychological tests. Cognitively impaired MS patients had a significant increase of θ power in the frontal regions and a diffuse decrease in coherence that were not found in cognitively intact patients. Moreover, coherence decrease, indicating involvement of functional corticocortical connections [47], was significantly correlated with brain MRI lesion load immediately underlying cortex. This finding is consistent with other MRI studies which demonstrated a significant correlation between the global cognitive impairment and the severity of white matter abnormalities of the hemispheres, of corpus callosum atrophy, and ventricular dilatation [41, 48-50]. Closer correlations have been found between cognitive impairment and both subcortical lesion load [39, 40] and corpus callosum atrophy [51]. Moreover, the analysis of regional cerebral lesion load showed significant relationships with specific cognitive functions [50-52]. Our EEG study [46] investigated patients with a progressive form of MS, in whom a higher prevalence of cognitive disturbances, compared to RRMS patients, has been reported [53, 54]. Interestingly, only SPMS patients had a significant increase of slow frequency of the frontal regions, while no significant change of EEG power was found in the PPMS group.

Another important neurophysiological test of brain function is the analysis of event-related potentials (ERPs), which are brain waves related to stimulus processing. P300, the most widely studied ERP, is a positive wave recorded over the scalp when subjects discriminate stimuli differing in respect of some physical dimension. P300 is thought to represent a closure of the evaluation process stimulus [55], and its latency has been proposed as an indicator of information processing speed [56]. This process is electively affected in MS [57] and, as a consequence, P300 latency is increased in MS patients [58]. The increase of P300 latency is correlated with the severity of cognitive impairment [59] and with the degree of white matter involvement [60]. In addition, ERPs secondary to specific cognitive tasks may be of help in assessing specific cognitive domains, such as abstract reasoning and memory, which are selectively impaired in MS [33]. Pelosi et al. [61] investigated visual and auditory ERPs elicited with the Sternberg paradigm [62], assessing working memory, in a group of patients with clinically isolated myelopathy suggestive of MS. The component of the response that has been shown to be sensitive to memory loading in healthy control subjects was affected in patients with memory dysfunction. Finally, simple and complex reaction times provide a parametric measure of speed of sensorimotor and cognitive processing, which revealed abnormalities in MS patients related to neuropsychological impairment [61, 63]; they might also be useful in the assessment of functional brain involvement in PPMS.

Future studies combining EEG/ERP functional investigation, MRI measures of brain damage, and neuropsychological assessment may help in clarifying to what extent the brain is involved in PPMS.

Conclusions

Standard EPs are easy to obtain in most neurophysiology laboratories, with only minor discomfort for the patients. In the past, their use in MS has been limited to diagnosis. In this context, studies specifically devoted to the investigation of PPMS are lacking. Nevertheless, a promising and valuable contribution of EPs in the study of patients with progressive MS might be their use in the assessment of disease severity. The evaluation of standard EPs has so far produced similar results in PPMS and SPMS patients, possibly because of similar involvement of the sensory and motor central nervous pathways in these two groups of patients. In this respect, neurophysiological techniques such as EEG and ERPs that provide a measure of the overall brain involvement, are likely to become a useful tool in the assessment of these patients.

Acknowledgements. This work was partially supported by a grant from the Italian Ministry of University and Technological Research (protocol 9906151218-001).

References

1. Nuwer MR, Packwood JW, Lawrence WM, Ellison GW (1987) Evoked potentials predict the clinical changes in a multiple sclerosis drug study. Neurology 37:1754-1761
2. Filippi M, Campi A, Mammi S et al (1995) Brain MRI and multimodal evoked potentials in benign and secondary multiple sclerosis. J Neurol Neurosurg Psychiatry 58: 31-37
3. Lassmann H, Wisniewski HM (1979) Chronic relapsing experimental allergic encephalomyelitis: clinicopathological comparison with multiple sclerosis. Arch Neurol 36:490-497
4. Trapp BD, Peterson J, Ransohoff RM et al (1998) Axonal transection in the lesions of multiple sclerosis. N Engl J Med 338:278-285
5. Scolding N, Franklin R (1998) Axon loss in multiple sclerosis. Lancet 352:340-341
6. Ritchie JM, Rogart RB (1977) Density of sodium channels in mammalian myelinated nerve fibers and nature of the axonal membrane under the myelin sheath. Proc Natl Acad Sci USA 74:211-215
7. McDonald WI (1963) The effects of experimental demyelination on conduction in peripheral nerve: a histological and electrophysiological study. II. Electrophysiological observations. Brain 86:501-524
8. McDonald WI, Sears TA (1979) The effects of experimental demyelination on conduction in the central nervous system. Brain 93:583-598
9. Rasminsky M, Sears TA (1972) Internodal conduction in undissected demyelinated fibres. J Physiol (Lond) 227:323-350
10. Moreau T, Coles A, Wing M et al (1996) Transient increase in symptoms associated with cytokine release in patients with multiple sclerosis. Brain 119:225-237
11. Koller H, Siebler M, Hartung HP (1997) Immunologically induced electrophysiological dysfunction: implications for inflammatory diseases of the CNS and PNS. Prog Neurobiol 52:1-26
12. McDonald WI (1977) Pathophysiology of conduction in central nerve fibers. In: Desmedt JE (ed) Visual evoked potentials in man: new developments. Clarendon Press, Oxford, pp 427-437
13. Emerson RG (1998) Evoked potentials in clinical trials for multiple sclerosis. J Clin Neurophysiol 15:109-116

14. Comi G, Leocani L, Medaglini S et al (1999) Measuring evoked responses in multiple sclerosis. Mult Scler 5:263-267
15. Bjartmar C, Trapp BD (2001) Axonal and neuronal degeneration in multiple sclerosis: mechanisms and functional consequences. Curr Opin Neurol 14:271-278
16. McGavern DB, Murray PD, Rivera-Quinones C et al (2000) Axonal loss results in spinal cord atrophy, electrophysiological abnormalities and neurological deficits following demyelination in a chronic inflammatory model of multiple sclerosis. Brain 123:519-531
17. Gronseth GS, Ashman EJ (2000) Practice parameter: the usefulness of evoked potentials in identifying clinically silent lesions in patients with suspected multiple sclerosis (an evidence-based review): report of the Quality Standards Subcommittee of the American Academy of Neurology. Neurology 54:1720-1725
18. Leocani L, Comi G (2000) Neurophysiological investigations in multiple sclerosis. Curr Opin Neurol 13:255-261
19. Facchetti D, Mai R, Micheli A et al (1997) Motor evoked potentials and disability in secondary progressive multiple sclerosis. Can J Neurol Sci 24:332-337
20. Kira J, Tobimatsu S, Goto I, Hasuo K (1993) Primary progressive versus relapsing remitting multiple sclerosis in Japanese patients: a combined clinical, magnetic resonance imaging and multimodality evoked potential study. J Neurol Sci 117:179-185
21. Andersson T, Persson A (1990) Reproducibility of somatosensory evoked potentials (SEPs) after median nerve stimulation. Electroencephalogr Clin Neurophysiol 30:205-211
22. Martinelli V, Comi G (1995) Il valore prognostico dei potenziali evocati nella sclerosi multipla. In: Comi G (ed) I potenziali evocati nella sclerosi multipla - diagnosi, prognosi e monitoraggio. Springer, Milan, pp 105-116
23. Ormerod IEC, Miller DH, McDonald WI et al (1987) The role of NMR imaging in the assessment of multiple sclerosis and isolated neurological lesions. A quantitative study. Brain 110:1579-1616
24. Andersson PB, Waubant E, Gee L, Goodkin DE (1999) Multiple sclerosis that is progressive from the time of onset: clinical characteristics and progression of disability. Arch Neurol 56:1138-1142
25. Kurtzke JF (1983) Rating neurological impairment in multiple sclerosis: an Expanded Disability Status Scale (EDSS). Neurology 33:1444-1452
26. Sater RA, Rostami AM, Galetta S et al (1999) Serial evoked potential studies and MRI imaging in chronic progressive multiple sclerosis. J Neurol Sci 171:79-83
27. O'Connor P, Marchetti P, Lee L, Perera M (1998) Evoked potential abnormality scores are a useful measure of disease burden in relapsing-remitting multiple sclerosis. Ann Neurol 44:404-407
28. Kidd D, Thompson PD, Day BL et al (1998) Central motor conduction time in progressive multiple sclerosis. Correlations with MRI and disease activity. Brain 121:1109-1116
29. Kalkers NF, Hintzen RQ, van Waesberghe JH et al (2001) Magnetization transfer histogram parameters reflect all dimensions of MS pathology, including atrophy. J Neurol Sci 184:155-162
30. van Walderveen MA, Lycklama A, Nijeholt GJ et al (2001) Hypointense lesions on T1-weighted spin-echo magnetic resonance imaging: relation to clinical characteristics in subgroups of patients with multiple sclerosis. Arch Neurol 58:76-81
31. Rovaris M, Bozzali M, Santuccio G et al (2000) Relative contributions of brain and cervical cord pathology to multiple sclerosis disability: a study with magnetisation transfer ratio histogram analysis. J Neurol Neurosurg Psychiatry 69:723-727
32. Comi G, Filippi M, Martinelli V et al (1995) Brain magnetic resonance imaging correlates of cognitive impairment in primary and secondary progressive multiple sclerosis. J Neurol Sci 132:222-227
33. Rao SM, Leo GJ, Bernardin L, Unverzagt F (1991) Cognitive dysfunction in multiple sclerosis. I. Frequency, patterns and predictions. Neurology 41:685-691

34. Peyser JM, Rao SM, Larocca NG, Kaplan E (1990) Guidelines for neuropsychological research in multiple sclerosis. Arch Neurol 47:94-97
35. Filley CM, Heaton RK, Nelson LM et al (1989) A comparison of dementia in Alzheimer's disease and multiple sclerosis. Arch Neurol 46:157-161
36. Comi G, Filippi M, Martinelli V et al (1993) Brain magnetic resonance imaging correlates of cognitive impairment in multiple sclerosis. J Neurol Sci 115:66-73
37. Rao SM (1990) Multiple sclerosis. In: Cummings JL (ed) Subcortical dementia. Oxford University Press, New York, pp 164-180
38. Mahler ME, Benson DF (1990) Cognitive dysfunction in multiple sclerosis: a subcortical dementia? In: Rao SM (ed) Neurobehavioral aspects of multiple sclerosis. Oxford University Press, New York, pp 88-101
39. Damian MS, Schilling G, Bachmann G et al (1994) White matter lesions and cognitive deficits: relevance of lesion pattern? Acta Neurol Scand 90:430-436
40. Miki Y, Grossman RI, Udupa JK et al (1998) Isolated U-fiber involvement in MS-preliminary observations. Neurology 50:1301-1306
41. Rao SM, Leo GJ, Haughton VM et al (1989) Correlation of magnetic resonance imaging with neuropsychological testing in multiple sclerosis. Neurology 39:161-166
42. Foong J, Rozewicz L, Chong WK et al (2000) A comparison of neuropsychological deficits in primary and secondary progressive multiple sclerosis. J Neurol 247:97-101
43. Comi G, Leocani L, Locatelli T et al (1999) Electrophysiological investigations in multiple sclerosis dementia. Electroencephalogr Clin Neurophysiol Suppl 50:480-485
44. Harrer G, Harrer H, Kofler B, Haas R (1985) Multiple sclerosis and the electroencephalogram (computer EEG studies). Wien Med Wochenschr 135:38-40
45. Locatelli T, Filippi M, Martinelli V et al (1993) EEG mapping in multiple sclerosis. Riv Neurobiol 39:233-237
46. Leocani L, Magnani G, Locatelli T et al (1998) EEG correlates of cognitive impairment in MS. Ital J Neurol Sci 19:S413-S417
47. Thatcher RW, Krause PJ, Hrybyk M (1986) Cortico-cortical associations and EEG coherence: a two-compartmental model. Electroencephalogr Clin Neurophysiol 64:123-143
48. Franklin GM, Nelson LM, Filter CM, Heaton RK (1989) Cognitive loss in multiple sclerosis. Arch Neurol 46:162-167
49. Comi G, Rovaris M, Falautano M et al (1999) A multiparametric MRI study of frontal lobe dementia in multiple sclerosis. J Neurol Sci 171:135-144
50. Swirsky-Sacchetti T, Mitchell DR, Seward J et al (1992) Neuropsychological and structural brain lesions in multiple sclerosis: a regional analysis. Neurology 42:1291-1295
51. Foong J, Rozewicz L, Quaghebeur G et al (1997) Executive functions in multiple sclerosis. The role of frontal lobe pathology. Brain 120:15-26
52. Rovaris M, Filippi M, Falautano M et al (1998) Relationship between MR abnormalities and patterns of cognitive impairment in multiple sclerosis. Neurology 50:1601-1608
53. Heaton RK, Nelson LM, Thompson DS et al (1985) Neuropsychological findings in relapsing-remitting and chronic-progressive multiple sclerosis. J Consult Clin Psychol 53:103-110
54. Beatty WW, Goodkin DE, Monson N, Beatty PA (1989) Cognitive disturbances in patients with relapsing remitting multiple sclerosis. Arch Neurol 46:1113-1119
55. Desmedt JE (1980) P300 in serial tasks: an essential post-decision closure mechanism. Prog Brain Res 54:682-686
56. Kutas M, McCarthy G, Donchin E (1977) Augmenting mental chronometry: the P300 as a measure of stimulus evaluation time. Science 197:792-795
57. Rao SM, Leo GJ, St Hubin Faubert P (1989) On the nature of memory disturbance in multiple sclerosis. J Clin Exp Neuropsychol 11:699-712
58. Newton MR, Barrett G, Callanan MM, Towell AD (1989) ERP P300 in multiple sclerosis. Brain 112:1636-1660

59. Giesser BS, Schroeder MM, LaRocca NG et al (1992) Endogenous event-related potentials as indices of dementia in multiple sclerosis patients. Electroencephalogr Clin Neurophysiol 82:320-329
60. Honig LS, Ramsay RE, Sheremata WA (1992) Event-related potentials P300 in multiple sclerosis. Relation to magnetic resonance imaging and cognitive impairment. Arch Neurol 49:44-50
61. Pelosi L, Geesken JM, Holly M et al (1997) Working memory impairment in early multiple sclerosis. Evidence from an event-related potential study of patients with clinically isolated myelopathy. Brain 120:2039-2058
62. Sternberg S (1966) High-speed scanning in human memory. Science 153:652-654
63. Leocani L, Magnani G, Locatelli T et al (1998) EEG correlates of cognitive impairment in MS. Ital J Neurol Sci 19:S413-S417

Chapter 5

Neuropsychology

M.P. AMATO

Introduction and Background

For the greater part of this century clinicians have grossly underestimated the importance of cognitive dysfunction in multiple sclerosis (MS); only during the last two decades have they become increasingly aware of the prevalence of MS-related cognitive impairment and its profound impact on function.

In the early 1980s, with the advent of magnetic resonance imaging (MRI), MS became particularly attractive to researchers as the prototypical subcortical, white-matter dementing disease: the result was a considerable amount of research in this area. Using formal neuropsyhological testing the prevalence of cognitive impairment in MS patients has been estimated at between 43% and 65% [1]. Kahana et al.'s [2] and Sheperd's [3] estimates of 7% and 25%, respectively, illustrate the reduced sensitivity of clinical as opposed to neuropsychological methods. Severe dementia is observed in approximately 20%-30% of cognitively impaired MS patients [1]. Cognitive dysfunction can have a dramatic impact on the everyday life and social functioning of MS patients, independently of the degree of physical disability. Cognitive impairment significantly affects the ability to maintain employment [4-6]; moreover, patients with cognitive impairment require greater personal assistance in carrying out daily living activities, and are less likely to engage in social activities than cognitively intact MS patients – findings which obtain even after controlling for severity of physical disability and disease course [4-6]. Finally, cognitive impairment can also limit the capacity of the patient to benefit from rehabilitation [7].

Only in the last few years have explorative studies focused specifically on the cognitive capacities and MRI findings of patients with primary progressive (PP)MS, to investigate whether neuropsychological findings in these patients may differ from those observed in patients with the secondary progressive (SP) form of the disease.

This chapter is divided into two sections. The first provides an overview of current knowledge about the pattern of cognitive dysfunction in MS, and its clinical and neuroimaging correlates. The second section reviews existing data on the neuropsychology of PPMS and discusses implications for future research in this area.

Overview

Pattern of Neuropsychological Dysfunction

The nature of MS-related cognitive impairment can make it difficult for the clinician to detect. It is typically circumscribed (i.e., limited to specific cognitive domains) rather than global, and pronounced aphasia-apraxia-agnosia syndrome, which might be readily recognized during everyday practice visits, occurs rarely. It has to be remembered, moreover, that there is considerable interpatient variability with regard to the pattern and severity of the deficits, while most of the neuropsychological investigations of MS patients are based on group studies which may mask these individual differences [1].

In regard to *general intelligence*, MS patients as a group display relatively small declines on standardized measures of intelligence. When a decline has been reported on the Wechsler scales it has been mainly related to the Performance IQ subscale, which can be negatively affected by motor or coordination problems [1].

Memory is the most extensively investigated cognitive function in MS patients. Short-term memory deficits, although present, are less marked than those affecting long-term memory. Both verbal and nonverbal memory are adversely affected, and the mechanism involves failure at both acquisition and retrieval stages: deficits are, however, more frequent on tests of recall than recognition [1]. Implicit memory, which relates to learning and remembering without conscious awareness, is largely spared [1]. Finally, the ability of MS patients to appraise their own memory (called metamemory), is generally compromised [8]. This implies that patients' self-reports about memory are likely to be inaccurate. Metamemory may be, in part, a function of the prefrontal cortex, and deficits in metamemory in one study [9] correlated with impairment in frontal lobe tasks. Finally, metamemory impairment seems to be related to the overall severity of cognitive dysfunction [10].

Reduced *speed of information processing* and impaired *attention* are hallmarks of cognitive dysfunction in MS. Attention is generally compromised before memory deficits appear: therefore, impaired attention can represent a sensitive indicator of incipient cognitive decline in MS patients [1].

Frontal lobe and executive functions are often impaired in MS. Executive functions are higher-level cognitive functions, which include abstract reasoning and concept formation, problem solving, planning, and self-monitoring. Executive dysfunction clearly affects performance on other cognitive and motor tasks [1]. It has been specifically associated with impairment on explicit memory tasks, as well as with failure to apply systematic strategies to facilitate learning and recall [11-13]. Interestingly, performance on measures of executive function can also predict the potential benefit from various programs of cognitive rehabilitation [13].

Language functions have received less attention than other aspects of cognitive decline in MS and have been considered to remain relatively intact. Frank abnormalities of language are rare, although case reports of MS patients with aphasia syndromes have been published [1]. Carefully conducted studies focusing on linguistic functions in MS patients [14-15] have shown their difficulties with tests of naming, reading, verbal fluency, and verbal comprehension. It has been hypothesized that such problems are not tied primarily to a breakdown of linguistic processes, but rather derive from damage to other cognitive faculties [1]. Thus, language impairment in MS may be more common than initially thought: language problems are likely to have important functional consequences, disrupting interpersonal relationships and affecting work performance.

Clinical Correlates

Studies of correlations between cognitive deficits and clinical variables have provided conflicting evidence [16-21]. Cognitive impairment tends to be more prevalent in the later stages of the disease, although it may be detectable as an initial presentation [22], during the early phase [6, 23-25], or in the presence of limited physical disability [6, 23-25]. With few exceptions [23, 26], duration of disease has not emerged as a contributory factor [4, 6, 16]. Disability level as measured on the Expanded Disability Status Scale (EDSS) [27] is generally a modest predictor of overall cognitive function [4, 20]; indeed, the EDSS is mainly weighted for ambulation and is clearly insensitive to cognitive decline [28]. Moreover, patients with prominent spinal cord involvement can have substantial physical disability while remaining cognitively intact. Specific neurological signs such as cerebellar or brainstem findings may have slightly better predictive value than overall EDSS [4]. In contrast, clinical progression of the disease clearly increases the probability of developing MS-related cognitive impairment [23, 29]. In one study [30], cognitive function appears to fluctuate in conjunction with disease relapses and remission phases, although these changes may not be uniform across all cognitive domains. The relationship between cognitive dysfunction and fatigue is under debate: a recent positron emission tomography (PET) study of MS patients with fatigue shows abnormal glucose metabolism in regions involved in key cognitive functions [31]. In general, depression correlates only weakly with overall cognitive function in MS patients [1].

Neuroimaging Correlates

Cognitive impairment in MS is more strongly associated with MRI parameters than it is with clinical characteristics. Contrary to early assertions that the majority of T2-visible lesions are "clinically silent," it is now recognized that these lesions can have substantial effects on cognitive function. Cross-sectional studies have found moderate to strong correlations between the degree of cognitive dysfunction and total cerebral lesion load on T2-weighted images [32-34]; in one study [32], a total lesion area of 30 cm² or more was an almost certain indicator of significant cognitive decline. Longitudinal studies have found even stronger correlations pointing to increasing lesion load in the brain as a critical determinant of a patient cognitive outcome [22, 23, 35, 36]. Cognitive dysfunction in MS has also been associated with atrophy of the corpus callosum [6, 33, 37], generalized brain atrophy [37-39], and extensive periventricular involvement [32, 37, 40, 41]. Attempts to relate the location of cerebral white matter lesions to specific patterns of cognitive test performance have provided conflicting results [1]. Several factors may account for this: first, MS is usually a widespread disease; second, T2-visible lesions are nonspecific, reflecting several different pathological processes (e.g., edema, inflammation, demyelination, and axonal loss) with different impacts on cognitive function; finally, performance on most neuropsychological tests probably reflects the activation of distributed cognitive networks rather than of a specific cerebral region.

Pathology visible on T2-weighted images, however, is not the only pathology in MS, and the focal effect of lesions is only a partial explanation of cognitive dysfunction. Neuropsychological test performance also correlates with T1-hypointense lesion burden [34] and N-acetylaspartate/creatine ratios determined through MR spectroscopy [42]. Moreover, magnetization transfer imaging (MTI), which is sensitive to demyelination and axonal damage, allows us to identify abnormalities in normal-appearing white matter (NAWM) that can contribute to cognitive impairment, particularly in patients with PPMS [34, 43].

Neuropsychology of PPMS

In the majority of the studies on cognitive impairment in MS the category "chronic progressive" MS includes both patients with the primary and those with the secondary progressive forms of the disease; only a few studies have assessed the frequency, severity, and pattern of cognitive dysfunction separately in these two groups of patients.

Cross-Sectional Studies

In many cross-sectional studies subjects with a chronic progressive (CP) course consistently perform worse on neuropsychological testing than do those with a relapsing-remitting (RR) course [19, 44-46]. The pattern of cognitive involvement in these patients is characterized mainly by deficits of attention and speed of information processing, memory, executive functions, and verbal fluency [47-49].

Heaton et al. [19] studied 100 patients with either RRMS or CPMS, who were consecutively admitted to a neurological ward, and a similar number of healthy controls. Both CP and RR patients were more cognitively impaired than the control group, and CP patients were, in turn, more cognitively impaired than RR patients on most cognitive measures. These differences did not correlate to greater sensory or motor impairment in the CP group and persisted after controlling for the duration of the disease (which was longer in the CP group). Rao et al. [50] confirmed this result, comparing the performance of RR and CP patients and a control group of subjects with back pain. While no difference was observed between the RR group and the control subjects, CP patients showed a significantly worse performance. A stepwise regression analysis showed that these differences were independent of physical disability and disease duration. Indirect evidence supporting disease course as an important predictor of cognitive dysfunction also comes from studies confined to one of the subgroups, showing that memory is significantly impaired in over half of patients with a CP course [1]. In contrast with these findings, Beatty et al. [51] examined 42 patients with an RR and 43 with a CP course, and using multiple regression techniques found that progressive course was an excellent predictor of physical disability but a weak predictor of performance on individual cognitive measures.

To date only two studies have attempted to compare the cognitive abilities of PP and SP patients. Matching these patients is problematic, as the groups inevitably differ either in levels of physical disability or disease duration.

Comi et al. [52] compared the neuropsychological performance and MRI findings of 14 patients with PPMS and 17 with SPMS. Patients with PPMS and SPMS had similar mean ages and degrees of disability, but significantly different durations of the disease. Patients were given tests exploring frontal functions/abstract reasoning, short-term memory, long-term memory, visuospatial skills, attention, and language. The results were considered abnormal when they differed by more than two standard deviations from the published norms for the healthy population, and patients were considered to be cognitively impaired when they failed at least three tests. Cognitive impairment was found in 9/17 (53%) patients with SPMS and in only 1/14 (7%) of those with PPMS. Moreover, only two patients with SPMS had normal results in all the tests, while 10 patients with PPMS did so. Using a grading system to quantify the MRI cerebral lesion load, the study found that patients with SPMS had higher total, periventricular, and nonperiventricular MRI lesion loads than patients with PPMS. In addition, patients with SPMS and neuropsychological deficits had higher nonperiventricular lesion loads than those with SPMS who were cognitively intact, whereas periventricular regions were involved to a similar degree in both groups. In particular, the frontal lobe was significantly more involved in the impaired group. The authors concluded that cognitive impairment is almost exclusive to patients with SPMS, whereas even subtle cognitive impairment seems to be very rare in patients with PPMS.

These results were not confirmed by Foong et al. [53]. These authors compared 13 PPMS and 12 SPMS patients with similar duration of the progressive phase and a comparable degree of physical disability on the EDSS. A battery of neuropsychological tests assessing attention and short-term and working memory was administered to the patients, and their performance was compared to that of 20 healthy controls matched for age and premorbid IQ. Total cerebral lesion load on T2-weighted MRI was also measured. Both PPMS and SPMS patients performed significantly worse than controls in most of the neuropsychological tests. Although the raw scores suggested that SP patients performed worse than PP patients in most of the neuropsychological tests, the difference reached statistical significance only for a spatial working memory task. There was also a little difference in the proportion of PP (6/13) versus SP (8/12) patients who had severe cognitive impairment. Finally, total lesion load was significantly higher in SP than in PP patients, although no significant correlations were found between total lesion load and any of the neuropsychological tests in either the PP or the SP group.

Some methodological differences may in part account for these differences. In the study by Comi et al. [52], the correction of scores for age and education according to published norms (rather than comparison with a concurrent control group) may have reduced the sensitivity in detecting cognitive dysfunction. Other problems are differences in the method of MRI assessment and different matching of the patients in terms of disease duration or duration of the progressive phase. Sampling differences or a chance effect due to the small numbers are also possible.

The largest study of the cognitive function of patients with PPMS has been carried out by Camp et al. [38]. This study assessed the neuropsychological performance and MRI aspects of PP and transitional progressive (TP) MS patients and provided evidence that cognitive impairment in PP patients is probably more common than was previously believed. Patients with TPMS have been shown to be clinically very similar to the PP group [54] and different from the group termed "progressive-relapsing" by Lublin and Reingold [55], in that they have a predominantly progressive course with only a single relapse. In this study, 63 patients (43 PP, 20 TP) were individually matched with healthy controls. These patients were taken from a larger cohort (158 PP, 33 TP) in which it had been demonstrated that there were no significant differences between the mean scores of the PP and TP groups on any of the cognitive variables. The neuropsychological assessment included Rao's Brief Repeatable Battery (BRB) [56], a reasoning test, and a measure of depression. Total brain T2 and T1-hypointense lesion loads were obtained for patients using a semiautomated contour technique. To allow broad comparison with Comi's data on cognitive impairment in PPMS, patients were considered to be cognitively impaired when they performed at least two standard deviations below the control mean on three or more subtests. The 63 patients performed significantly worse than controls in tests of verbal memory, attention, verbal fluency, and spatial reasoning, while showing relative preservation of verbal reasoning. The incidence of cognitive impairment was 28.6%, compared with the 7% previously reported by Comi et al. The demographic and clinical characteristics of the patients in these two studies were similar. An impairment index was constructed and applied to the patient data. This correlated moderately with T2 lesion load, T1-hypointense lesion load, and cerebral volume. Specifically, the MRI measures of T2 lesion load and T1-hypointense lesion load correlated better with impairment on the BRB, while the measure of cerebral volume showed a higher correlation with impairment on the abstract reasoning task. As in other reports [57], patients in this study had relatively low lesion loads on MRI.

Longitudinal Studies

Results obtained from the few studies that have examined the evolution of cognitive functioning in MS are controversial. Both cognitive preservation [35, 36, 58, 59] and progressive deterioration [6, 22, 60] have been reported, and remarkable fluctuations have been noted during very brief follow-up periods [23]. In these studies PP and SP patients have been included in the "chronic progressive" category, and so far no longitudinal study has specifically assessed the evolution of cognitive performance in patients with PPMS. Some of these studies, however, provide indirect evidence that the evolution of cognitive dysfunction in the two groups is not strikingly different. Hohol et al. [35] followed up 44 patients for one year, eight of whom had a PP and five an SP course. Overall, there was no decline in mean cognitive performance measured on the BRB. There were significant correlations between test performance and total brain lesion load and brain atrophy at MRI. Moreover, there were no significant differences in mean baseline performances or changes over time for any of the subjects among patients with PP or SP disease course. Kujala et al. [60] have followed up over three years the evolution of cognitive performances in two clinically and demographically similar MS groups, 20 "cognitively preserved" and 22 "cognitively mildly deteriorated" patients, and in 34 healthy controls, using an extensive neuropsychological test battery sensitive to mild cognitive deterioration. The "cognitively preserved" group showed substantial stability over the follow-up period, whereas the initially "mildly deteriorated" group demonstrated progressive cognitive decline on many tests, suggesting that incipient cognitive decline may be widespread and progressive in nature. No statistically significant differences between the patient groups were observed at baseline: preserved: 5 RR/8 PP/7 SP; deteriorated: 1 RR/13 PP/8 SP. Moreover, at the end of the follow-up period, patients with SPMS did not exhibit more cognitive deterioration than patients with PPMS.

Amato et al. have published the results of a 10-year study on the cognitive performance of 50 patients with early-onset MS and 70 healthy controls [6, 29], whose cognitive capacities were assessed by means of tests of long-term and short-term memory, visuospatial abilities, abstract reasoning, verbal fluency, and language. At the end of the follow-up period the study group included five PP and 14 SP patients. The study shows that with time the likelihood increases that subjects who do not have cognitive impairment may deteriorate: only 20 of the 37 patients in this sample who did not have cognitive impairment on initial testing remained unchanged by the end of the follow-up, when the proportion of subjects who were cognitively impaired reached 56% (Table 1). Degree of physical disability, progressive disease course, and increasing age were independent predictors of

Table 1. Evolution of cognitive dysfunction in MS patients

No. of failed subtests	First testing	No. of patients Second testing	Third testing
0 - 2 (no impairment)	37/50 (74%)	25/49 (51%)	20/45 (44%)
3-5 (mild impairment)	4/50 (8%)	16/49 (33%)	15/45 (34%)
> 5 (moderate impairment)	9/50 (18%)	8/49 (16%)	10/45 (22%)

Table 2. Multiple linear regression analysis: Predictors of cognitive performance (number of failed subtests in the MS group)

Significant predictors	r (p)	R^2
EDSS	1.36 (0.001)	
Progressive course	0.96 (0.014)	0,51
Age	0.33 (0.010)	

a poor cognitive outcome. There were no significant differences in the cognitive performance of PP and SP patients at the end of the follow-up period (Table 2).

Conclusions

There is a dearth of research focusing on the cognitive capacities of patients with PPMS. Some limitations of published studies, such as the small sample sizes, render it difficult to draw any firm conclusion on whether PPMS and SPMS patients are characterized by differing frequency and severity of cognitive dysfunction. The pattern of cognitive dysfunction in PP patients seems to be similar to that previously reported, with a relative sparing of verbal reasoning in one study.

Some cross-sectional studies have contradicted the paradigm that in patients with a PP disease course, as opposed to SP patients, cognitive impairment is rare and generally not severe, possibly due to the prominent involvement at the spinal cord rather than at the cerebral level; longitudinal studies have pointed to a similar conclusion. In one of these studies, the prevalence of cognitive dysfunction in PPMS was estimated at around 28%; in another study, when the duration of the progressive phase was taken into account as a matching criterion, the frequency and severity of cognitive impairment was similar in PP and SP patients.

Another issue is whether the pathophysiological mechanisms of cognitive dysfunction in PPMS and SPMS may be different. Both cross-sectional and longitudinal studies point to the importance of MRI cerebral lesion load as a critical determinant of a patient's cognitive performance. Although PP patients have significantly lower total brain lesion loads than SP patients, their physical disability and cognitive deficits seem not to be strikingly different. This suggests that cognitive dysfunction in PPMS patients may have a complex and multifactorial origin. In particular, on conventional MRI, detectable lesions in these groups may differ in terms of the severity of axonal loss, demyelination, and gliosis, with differing impact on cognitive function. Moreover, microscopic abnormalities in the NAWM can contribute to cognitive dysfunction in these patients.

Finally, the integrity of cortical tracts is another issue hardly addressed by conventional MRI, a factor to be taken into account since both white and gray matter are involved in the disease process. Newer imaging techniques, particularly those examining NAWM and the cortex, as well as longitudinal studies will provide further insights on this topic.

References

1. Rao SM (1997) Neuropsychological aspects of multiple sclerosis. In: Raine CS, McFarland HF, Tourtellotte WW (eds) Multiple sclerosis: clinical and pathogenetic basis. London, Chapman & Hall, London, pp 357-362
2. Kahana EK, Leibovitz U, Alter M (1971) Cerebral multiple sclerosis. Neurology 21:1179-1185
3. Sheperd D (1987) Memory and brain. Oxford University Press, New York
4. Rao SM, Leo GJ, Ellington L et al (1991) Cognitive dysfunction in MS: II: Impact on employment and social functioning. Neurology 41:692-696
5. Beatty WW, Blanco CR, Wilbanks SL et al (1995) Demographic, clinical, and cognitive characteristics of MS patients who continue to work. J Neurol Rehab 9:167-173
6. Amato MP, Ponziani G, Pracucci G et al (1995) Cognitive impairment in early-onset multiple sclerosis: pattern, predictors, and impact on everyday life in a 4-year follow-up. Arch Neurol 52:168-172
7. Langdon DW, Thompson AJ (1999) Multiple sclerosis: a preliminary study of selected variables affecting rehabilitation outcome. Mult Scler 5:94-100
8. Beatty WW, Monson N (1991) Metamemory in MS. J Clin Expl Neuropsychol 13:309-327
9. Taylor R (1990) Relationships between cognitive test performance and everyday cognitive difficulties in MS. Br J Clin Psychol 29:251-252
10. Kujala P, Portin R, Ruutianen J (1996) Memory deficits and early cognitive deterioration in multiple sclerosis. Acta Neurol Scand 93:329-335
11. Troyer AK, Fisk JD, Archibald CJ et al (1996) Conceptual reasoning as a mediator of verbal recall in patients with multiple sclerosis. J Clin Exp Neuropsychol 18:211-219
12. Arnett PA, Rao SM, Grafman M et al (1997) Executive functions in multiple sclerosis: analysis of temporal ordering, semantic encoding, and planning abilities. Neuropsychology 11:535-544
13. Canellopoulou M, Richardson JTE (1998) The role of executive function in imagery mnemonics: evidence from multiple sclerosis. Neuropsychology 36:1181-1188
14. Friend KB, Rabin BM, Groninger L, Deluty RH, Bever C, Grattan L (1999) Language functions in patients with multiple sclerosis. Clin Neuropsychol 13:78-94
15. Kujala P, Portin R, Ruutiainen J (1996) Language functions in incipient cognitive decline in multiple sclerosis. J Neurol Sci 141:79-86
16. Ivnik RJ (1978) Neuropsychological test performance as a function of the duration of MS-related symptomatology. J Clin Psychiatry 39:304-307
17. Marsh GG (1980) Disability and intellectual function in multiple sclerosis. J Nerv Ment Dis 168:758-762
18. Rao SM, Glatt S, Hammeke TA et al (1985) Chronic progressive multiple sclerosis: relationship between cerebral ventricular size and neuropsychological impairment. Arch Neurol 42:678-682
19. Heaton RK, Nelson LM, Thompson DS et al (1985) Neuropsychological findings in relapsing-remitting and chronic-progressive multiple sclerosis. J Consult Clin Psychol 53:103-110
20. Rao SM, Hammeke TA, McQuillen MP et al (1984) Memory disturbance in chronic-progressive multiple sclerosis. Arch Neurol 41:625-631
21. Thornton AE, Raz N (1977) Memory impairment in multiple sclerosis: a quantitative review. Neuropsychology 11:357-366
22. Feinstein A, Kartsounis LD, Miller DH et al (1992) Clinically isolated lesions of the

type seen in multiple sclerosis: a cognitive, psychiatric, and MRI follow-up study. J Neurol Neurosurg Psychiatry 55:869-876

23. Feinstein A, Ron M, Thompson A (1993) A serial study of psychometric and magnetic resonance imaging changes in multiple sclerosis. Brain 116:569-602

24. Lyon-Caen O, Jouvent R, Hauser S et al (1986) Cognitive function in recent-onset demyelinating diseases. Arch Neurol 43:1138-1141

25. Grant CM, McDonald WI, Trimble MR et al (1984) Deficient learning and memory in early and middle phases of multiple sclerosis. J Neurol Neurosurg Psychiatry 47:250-255

26. McIntosh-Michaelis SA, Roberts MH, Wilkinson SM et al (1991) The prevalence of cognitive impairment in a community survey of multiple sclerosis. Br J Clin Psychol 30:333-348

27. Kurtzke JF (1983) Rating neurological impairment in multiple sclerosis: an expanded disability status scale (EDSS). Neurology 33:1444-1452

28. Amato MP, Ponziani G (1999) Quantification of impairment in MS: discussion of the scales in use. Mult Scler 5:216-219

29. Amato MP, Ponziani G, Siracusa G, Sorbi S (2001) Cognitive dysfunction in early-onset multiple sclerosis. A reappraisal after 10 years. Arch Neurol 58:1602-1606

30. Foong J, Rozewicz L, Queghebeur G et al (1998) Neuropsychology deficits in multiple sclerosis after an acute relapse. J Neurol Neurosurg Psychiatry 64:529-532

31. Roelcke U, Kappos L, Lechner-Scott J et al (1997) Reduced glucose metabolism in the frontal cortex and basal ganglia of multiple sclerosis patients with fatigue: a ^{18}F-fluorodeoxyglucose positron emission tomography study. Neurology 48:1566-1571

32. Rao SM, Leo GJ, Haughton VM et al (1989) Correlation of magnetic resonance imaging with neuropsychological testing in multiple sclerosis. Neurology 39:161-166

33. Huber SJ, Bornstein RA, Rammohan KW et al (1997) Magnetic resonance imaging correlates of neuropsychological impairment analysis in multiple sclerosis. Arch Neurol 54:1018-1025

34. Rovaris M, Filippi M, Falautano M et al (1998) Relation between MR abnormalities and patterns of cognitive impairment in multiple sclerosis. Neurology 6:1601-1608

35. Hohol MJ, Guttmann CRG, Orav J et al (1997) Serial neuropsychological assessment and magnetic resonance imaging analysis in multiple sclerosis. Arch Neurol 54:1018-1025

36. Mariani C, Farina E, Cappa SF et al (1991) Neuropsychological assessment in multiple sclerosis: a follow-up study with magnetic resonance imaging. J Neurol 238:395-400

37. Comi G, Filippi M, Martinelli V et al (1993) Brain magnetic resonance imaging correlates of cognitive impairment in multiple sclerosis. J Neurol Sci 115(Suppl):S66-S73

38. Camp SJ, Stevenson VL, Thompson AJ et al (1999) Cognitive function in primary progressive and transitional progressive multiple sclerosis: a controlled study with MRI correlates. Brain 122:1341-1348

39. Clark CM, James G, Li D et al (1992) Ventricular size, cognitive function and depression in patients with multiple sclerosis. Can J Neurol Sci 19:352-356

40. Anzola GP, Bevilacqua L, Cappa SF et al (1990) Neuropsychological assessment in patients with relapsing-remitting multiple sclerosis and mild functional impairment : correlation with magnetic resonance imaging. J Neurol Neurosurg Psychiatry 53:142-145

41. Maurelli M, Marchioni E, Cerretano R et al (1992) Neuropsychological assessment in MS: clinical, neurophysiological and neuroradiological relationships. Acta Neurol Scand 86:124-128

42. Foong J, Rozewicz L, Davie CA et al (1999) Correlates of executive function in multiple sclerosis: the use of magnetic resonance spectroscopy as an index of focal pathology. J Neuropsychiatry Clin Neurosci 11:45-50

43. Filippi M, Tortorella C, Rovaris M et al (2000) Changes in the normal appearing brain

tissue and cognitive impairment in multiple sclerosis. J Neurol Neurosurg Psychiatry 68:157-161

44. Minden SL, Moes EJ, Orav J et al (1990) Memory impairment in multiple sclerosis. J Clin Exp Neuropsychol 11:566-586

45. Grossman M, Armstrong C, Onishi K et al (1994) Patterns of cognitive impairment in relapsing-remitting and chronic-progressive multiple sclerosis. Neuropsychiatry Neuropsychol Behav Neurol 7:194-210

46. Filippi M, Alberoni M, Martinelli V et al (1994) Influence of clinical variables on neuropsychological performance in multiple sclerosis. Eur Neurol 34:324-328

47. Nocentini U, Rossini PM, Carlesimo GA et al (2001) Patterns of cognitive impairment in secondary progressive stable phase of multiple sclerosis: correlations with MRI findings. Eur Neurol 45:11-18

48. Beatty WW, Goodkin DE, Beatty PA, Monson N (1989) Frontal lobe dysfunction and memory impairment in patients with chronic progressive multiple sclerosis. Brain Cogn 11:73-86

49. Grigsby J, Ayarbe SD, Kravcisin N, Busenbark D (1994) Working memory impairment among persons with chronic progressive multiple sclerosis. J Neurol 241:125-131

50. Rao SM, Hammeke TA, Speech TJ (1987) Winsconsin Card Sort Test performance in relapsing-remitting and chronic-progressive multiple sclerosis. J Consult Clin Psychol 55:263-265

51. Beatty WW, Goodkin DE, Hertsgaard D, Monson N (1990b) Clinical and demographic predictors of cognitive performance in MS. Do diagnostic type, disease duration and disability matter? Arch Neurol 47:305-308

52. Comi G, Filippi M, Martinelli V et al (1995) Brain MRI correlates of cognitive impairment in primary and secondary progressive multiple sclerosis. J Neurol Sci 132:222-227

53. Foong J, Rozewicz L, Chong WK et al (2000) A comparison of neuropsychological deficits in primary and secondary progressive multiple sclerosis. J Neurol 247:97-101

54. Stevenson VL, Miller DH, Rovaris M et al (1999) Primary progressive and transitional progressive multiple sclerosis: a clinical and MRI cross sectional study. Neurology 52:839-845

55. Lublin FD, Reingold SC (1996) Defining the clinical course of multiple sclerosis: results of an international survey. Neurology 46:907-911

56. Rao SM (1990) Cognitive function study group, NMSS. A manual for the Brief Repeatable Battery of neuropsychological tests in multiple sclerosis. National Multiple Sclerosis Society, New York

57. Kidd D, Thorpe JW, Kendall BE et al (1996) MRI dynamics of brain and spinal cord in progressive multiple sclerosis. J Neurol Neurosurg Psychiatry 60:15-19

58. Jennekens-Schinkel A, La Boyrie PM, Lanser JBK et al (1990) Cognition in patients with multiple sclerosis after four years. J Neurol Sci 99:229-247

59. Patti F, Failla G, Ciancio MR et al (1998) Neuropsychological, neuroradiological and clinical findings in multiple sclerosis: a 3-year follow-up study. Eur J Neurol 5:283-286

60. Kujala P, Portin R, Ruutiainen J (1997) The progress of cognitive decline in multiple sclerosis: a controlled 3-year follow-up. Brain 120:289-297

Chapter 6

Overview of Treatment Trials: Early Baseline Clinical and MRI Data of the PROMiSe Trial

J.S. Wolinsky, P.A. Narayana, R. He

Introduction

Primary progressive multiple sclerosis (PPMS) is the least common clinical disease phenotype exhibited by MS patients. Current international consensus definitions of the various disease phenotypes demand that patients with PPMS have a progressive disease from onset and a clinical course without discernible attacks [1]. Some minor amount of improvement or worsening is allowed, but episodes that fit most modern trial definitions of acute relapses eliminate patients from this subtype and consign them to either secondary progressive or progressive relapsing MS categories, depending upon whether the attack occurred prior to or following the onset of their progressive neurologic dysfunction. Approximately 15% of MS patients have a progressive disease at onset, but nearly one-third of these will experience a clinical relapse. Thus, only 10% of all MS patients have PPMS. It is likely that some of these patients fail to recall remote episodes of neurologic dysfunction that may or may not have been attended by physicians or resulted in a formal diagnosis. Such cases of cryptic secondary progressive or "transitional" MS [2] may contaminate to some extent any cohort of rigorously defined PPMS patients. Further complicating our understanding of this clinical phenotype is the common use of the term "chronic progressive MS" to describe patient cohorts with secondary progressive, progressive relapsing, or PPMS.

Until recently, few investigators attempted specifically to isolate patients with PPMS for the purpose of clinical trials of therapeutic agents. Nor had generally accepted criteria for the clinical diagnosis of MS addressed the special issues raised by this phenotype [3]. However, apparent differences between the effects of various preparations of interferon-β in patients with relapsing and secondary progressive disease have recently highlighted the difficulties in separating the effects of therapeutic agents on disease progression from their benefits on attacks and the

Note: The PROMiSE Study Group dedicated this paper to two of its recently departed members, Dr. John Trotter, whose work on proteolipid protein opened our vision to a broader spectrum of organ-specific autoantigens that might be critical to the immunopathogenesis of MS, and Dr. John Whitaker who helped us to understand the importance of biomarkers to monitor the disease and direct the design of therapeutic trials. Their wisdom, guidance and personal grace will be deeply missed.

more inflammatory aspects of the underlying pathology as monitored by magnetic resonance imaging (MRI) [4, 5]. Treatment trials directed at patients with PPMS provide the ideal study population in which to investigate the effects of a therapeutic agent on clinical disease progression in the absence of the confounding influence of clinical attacks. However, studies of this MS phenotype introduce complexities of trial design not encountered in relapsing MS patient populations. This paper will concentrate on those issues of trial design specific to the study of PPMS as encountered in the development of the PROMiSe Trial, a multinational, multicenter, double-blind, placebo-controlled study to evaluate the efficacy, tolerability, and safety of glatiramer acetate for injection in PPMS patients.

Trial Design

Central to the issue of trial design is determining a reasonable primary objective. In this study we sought to determine whether glatiramer acetate could slow the progressive accumulation of disability in MS independent of its effects on relapses. For the above-mentioned reasons we felt that this issue could be best addressed in patients with PPMS. While some patients selected for clinical trials based on the PPMS phenotype could have one or more attacks on study to declare them as having progressive relapsing disease, the proportion of PPMS patients having such conversion on study should be small and not drive the results of an analysis of the primary efficacy end point. It was also assumed that, in the absence of relapses, a change in the Expanded Disability Status Scale (EDSS) score [6] sustained for at least 3 months would be a reasonable measure of clinical disease progression that would be unlikely to revert in this patient cohort. Therefore, the time to confirmed disease progression of an increase of one point in EDSS score sustained for at least 3 months for patients with a baseline EDSS score of 3.0-5.0, or an increase of at least 0.5 in this scale similarly sustained for patients with a baseline EDSS score of 5.5-6.5, was chosen as the primary efficacy end point of the trial.

Sample size projections were then constructed on the basis of available natural history data. These simulations were performed under the assumption that 40% of the enrolled patients would have an entry EDSS score of 3.0-5.0 (stratum I), and 60% would enroll with higher EDSS scores of 5.5-6.5 (stratum II). On the basis of natural history data [7], 50% of PPMS subjects in stratum I were expected to progress each year compared to 20% of those in stratum II. Figure 1 shows the results of these projections under the assumption of a 40% dropout rate for several different therapeutic effect sizes. Other simulations based on assumptions of smaller dropout rates had relatively little effect on the shape of the power curves. This is because of the time-to-event nature of the planned analysis of the primary outcome measure, where patients who are lost to follow-up are censored at the time of their last available visit. However, secondary outcome measures that are intention-to-treat-based remain quite sensitive to data loss from patient failure to complete the protocol.

A 40% effect and a 2:1 randomization of patients to active drug versus placebo

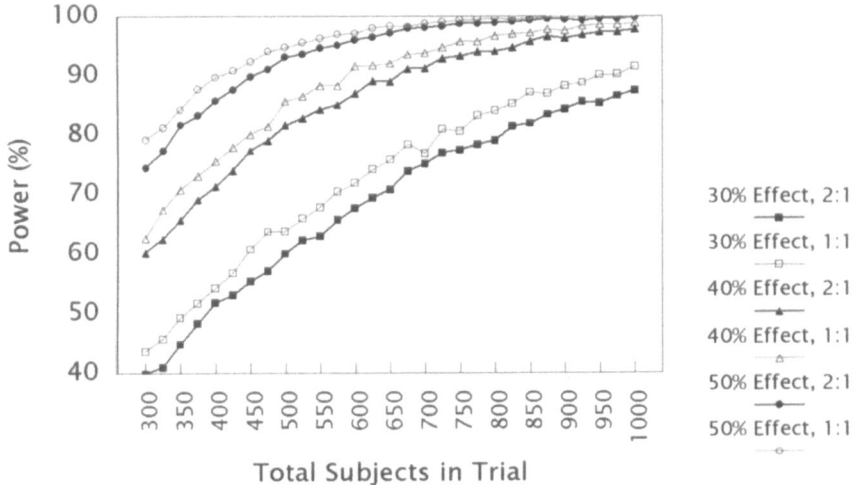

Fig. 1. Sample size simulations to achieve an overall α = 0.05 for an analysis of time to a predefined amount of progression from entry EDSS sustained for 3 months for patients randomized between two EDSS strata. Each curve represents a treatment effect size from 30% to 50% for either equal randomization between active drug and placebo or with unbalanced randomization at a 2:1 ratio as shown in the legend within the figure

set the targeted number of patients to be enrolled at 900 in a well-powered study. In actuality 943 patients were randomized by stratum and received at least one dose of study medication over 17 months, with enrollment closed in October 2000. In considering the results of other studies or in planning future trials in PPMS, it is worth noting that the sample size projections displayed in Fig. 1 demonstrate that at least 300 patients are required to show a 50% drug effect with patients equally randomized between active treatment and placebo in the trial with a minimal power of β equal to 0.8. These sample size simulations provide similar patient requirements to those derived from the Canadian natural history data [8], when one considers the allowance made for dropouts in the current projections.

Bornstein and his colleagues previously studied glatiramer acetate in a 2-year study of 106 patients with chronic progressive MS [9]. The study failed to meet predetermined efficacy criteria, although several posthoc analyses suggested a possible beneficial drug effect. Review of the case report forms from that study identified 30 patients either with PPMS (23 subjects) or whose disease was characterized by the onset of progressive gait disturbance more than 10 years after a single attack (transitional progressive MS). Using outcome measures and analytic techniques to be applied in the PROMiSe Trial to model the outcome of those 30 patients from the Bornstein study, trends were found that support the assumption of a delay in the time to progression and proportion of progression-free patients among the subjects randomized to glatiramer acetate.

A functional definition of PPMS was developed for the purposes of this trial.

To be eligible for study entry, all patients were required to have progressive neurologic symptoms including evidence of myelopathy for at least 6 months prior to the screening visit, leading the participating site's principal investigator to conclude that the patient had PPMS. Patients with a history of prior attacks of neurologic disease were specifically excluded. Objective evidence of pyramidal damage on neurologic examination was required, including a functional system score for the pyramidal system of at least 2. All patients were to have evidence of multilevel (disseminated) central nervous system disease based on objective evidence of neurologic examination alone or as supplemented by findings on MRI or visual or auditory evoked responses. Cervical spondylitic myelopathy had to be actively excluded by evidence of previous cervical imaging, preferably cervical MRI. Major competing causes of progressive neurologic disease including thyroid dysfunction, alterations of vitamin B_{12} metabolism, neurosyphilis, HTLV-I seropositivity, and Lyme disease needed to be excluded. Patients were to be between 30 and 65 years of age with an entry EDSS score of 3.0-6.5 inclusive.

All inclusion and exclusion criteria were addressed in an 18-point checklist. If all categories were checked in the affirmative, the site principal investigator was allowed to enter the patient into the study. Any patient who could not fulfill all 18 points required detailed review by a central patient eligibility committee. An important component of the eligibility criteria checklist was the documentation of the presence of cerebrospinal fluid (CSF) oligoclonal bands, an elevated IgG index, or an elevated IgG synthetic rate. While this was not an absolute requirement for study entry, the patient eligibility committee critically reviewed all patients lacking evidence of intrathecal synthesis of immunoglobulins for consistency with a diagnosis of PPMS. These definitions appeared consistent with approaches taken by others in defining cohorts of patients with PPMS for natural history studies [10]. However, as discussed further below, these criteria may not be as stringent as those of several recently proposed approaches for the diagnosis of PPMS [11, 12].

Clinical Demographics and Selected MRI Metrics at Entry

Not all of the clinical demographics, laboratory, and MRI data obtained at entry were available for all subjects at the time of preparation of this manuscript. Therefore, the number of patients for which different aspects of the data are displayed varies in the presentation that follows. A more complete, formal presentation of the entry data will be made in a future communication. Nonetheless, data from considerable numbers of subjects are available for most of the information presented that are likely to be highly representative of the final data tabulation. The clinical characteristics of patients entered into the study are shown in Table 1. Like other smaller cohorts of PPMS patients reported in the literature [8, 10, 13, 14], the patients in the PROMiSe Trial have a higher proportion of males, are older, and have a later age at onset and diagnosis than relapsing cohorts.

MRI was performed at baseline on all randomized patients using previously

Table 1. Clinical demographics at entry ($n = 943$)

Male	48.7%
White	89.8%
Age (years)	50.4 ± 8.3
Time since first symptom (years)	10.9 ± 7.5
Time since diagnosis	5.0 ± 5.1
Pyramidal FS score	3.0 ± 0.6
Cerebellar FS score	2.4 ± 2.0
Brainstem FS score	0.9 ± 1.0
Sensory FS score	1.8 ± 1.1
Bowel/Bladder FS score	1.6 ± 1.0
Visual FS score	1.1 ± 1.1
Mental FS score	0.7 ± 1.0
EDSS	4.9 ± 1.2
Ambulation index	3.1 ± 1.5
25-ft (7.5-m) timed walk (s)	12.2 ± 13.2
9-hole peg test (s)	30.2 ± 17.2
PASAT 2	38.9 ± 12.8
PASAT 3	48.4 ± 11.9
CSF positive	79.0%

FS, function system; *EDSS*, Expanded Dysability Status Scale; *PASAT*, Paced Auditory Serial Addition Test

detailed specialized pulse acquisition sequences [15]. These images were initially processed using previously defined automated segmentation strategies [16, 17]. This allowed us to compare selected MRI metrics obtained in patients with PPMS with those obtained in a different patient population at entry into another trial that used the same image acquisition and analysis strategy [18]. In that study, patients were selected across an identical EDSS range and all patients were classified according to disease type as either having relapsing or secondary progressive disease with or without continued attacks. A comparison of those patients with the first 534 patients entered into the PROMiSe trial is displayed in Table 2.

As suggested by others studying smaller PPMS cohorts [19], patients with PPMS are less likely to show gadolinium enhancement, as implied by their very low mean enhanced tissue volumes compared to patients with either relapsing or secondary progressive disease. The PPMS patients also have substantially reduced plaque burdens as measured on T2-weighted images when compared with relapsing patient cohorts of similar clinical disability [2]. In contrast, the hypointense lesion load seen on T1-weighted images of the PPMS group was rather similar to that observed in the comparative patients with secondary progressive disease, and substantially larger than that seen in patients with relapsing disease. At least among these comparably imaged and analyzed groups, the PPMS phenotype had a higher T1 hypointense lesion load as a proportion of their T2-defined disease burden than did those with relapsing or secondary progressive clinical disease phenotypes. This finding suggests that, while inflammatory lesions are less common among PPMS patients, they may result in proportionately greater tissue destruction over time than do those encountered in patients with relapsing forms

Table 2. Comparison of MRI metrics between clinical disease phenotypes

	RR ($n = 92$)	SP ($n = 626$)	SP with ($n = 346$)	SP without ($n = 280$)	PPMS ($n = 534$)
Gd (ml)[a]	0.4 ± 1.1	0.2 ± 0.8	0.2 ± 1.0	0.1 ± 2.6	0.04 ± 0.13
T2 BOD (ml)[b]	15.4 ± 12.7	16.5 ± 14.3	17.3 ± 15.4	15.6 ± 12.7	11.7 ± 14.9
T1 BOD (ml)[c]	0.5 ± 0.9	1.0 ± 2.4	1.0 ± 2.3	1.0 ± 2.6	0.8 ± 2.3
nCSF (%)[d]	17.1 ± 5.0	17.8 ± 5.1	17.8 ± 5.2	17.8 ± 5.0	15.8 ± 5.1
Z4[e]	0.5 ± 2.9	0.6 ± 2.8	0.7 ± 2.9	0.5 ± 2.7	−0.8 ± 2.7

RR, relapsing-remitting; *SP*, secondary progressive; *SP with*, SP with continued attacks; *SP without*, SP without continued attacks prior to entry into the trial; *PPMS*, primary progressive MS
[a] Mean volume in milliliters (± SD) of gadolinium-enhanced tissue
[b] Mean volume of plaque as determined by automated segmentation analysis from the AFFIRMATIVE images
[c] Hypointense lesion volume as determined from the post-gadolinium T1-weighted images by computer-assisted methods
[d] Intracranial tissue component segmented as cerebral spinal fluid (CSF) as a proportion of total segmented intracranial tissue contents
[e] An unweighted composite of the previous four MRI metrics

of the disease. Perhaps surprisingly, atrophy as measured by larger proportional intracranial CSF volumes was less prominent among the PPMS patients than among those with either secondary progressive or relapsing disease. The Z4 composite score should be close to zero for those subjects whose unweighted MRI metrics were most indicative of the average of the overall patient population, should become more positive for those patients whose overall MRI metrics indicate the most severe disease, and should be negative for those patients with the least pathologic change as measured by MRI [17]. Across the 1252 subjects studied, the Z4 scores by clinical phenotype clearly separated the PPMS subjects as those having the most "favorable" MRI metrics (Table 2).

New Segmentation Methodology for MRI Metric Determination

During the course of enrollment of patients into the trial, General Electric introduced a major machine upgrade. Images obtained with AFFIRMATIVE pulse sequences on these machines could no longer be segmented in a compatible fashion using our previously described image analysis algorithm. In order to obtain reliable and internally consistent data across both major General Electric 1.5-T machine types (5.x and LX platforms), our image analysis strategy and segmentation algorithms were revised. This process did not introduce important differences in the image acquisition protocol at the sites, except as required for the application of the AFFIRMATIVE sequence dictated by the two machine platforms. Previous postacquisition processing steps included anisotropic diffusion filtering, removal of extrameningeal tissue, radiofrequency inhomogeneity correction and intensity normalization, and 3D registration to a standard coordinate system prior to multispectral image segmentation that included information from 3D phase-contrast flow imaging and a step for automated removal of residual flow artifacts [15-17].

The new postacquisition processing steps incorporate radiofrequency inhomogeneity correction, removal of extrameningeal tissue and registration to a standard coordinate system, and, finally, spatial normalization. This strategy provides images that segment well and the same way whether obtained on 5.x or LX platforms. The automated segmentation algorithm was altered to accommodate the new postprocessed images and also to improve the quality of segmentation by introducing changes based on our experience with our previously published approach. The steps involved in the automated segmentation of the postprocessed images are shown in Fig. 2. Parzen maps based on various combinations of the postprocessed AFFIRMATIVE images were generated only once. The same maps

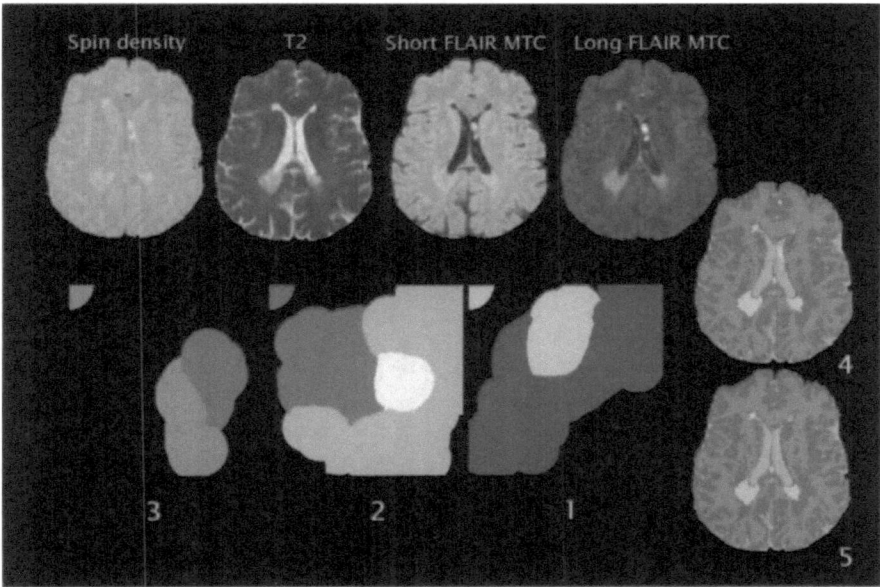

Fig. 2. Strategy for automated segmentation and tissue types based on a fully processed AFFIRMATIVE image set. The four images of a single 3-mm transaxial slice obtained with the AFFIRMATIVE pulse sequence are displayed in the *top row* of images in this figure. Short echo and long echo FLAIR MTC images are used to generate a Parzen map (*1*) for segmenting images as either BOD1 type lesion (*yellow*) or nonlesion intracranial tissue (*red*). Short echo FLAIR MTC and T2-weighted images are used to generate Parzen map (*2*) to classify BOD2 type lesion (*white*), CSF (*blue*), or other tissue (*gray*). Spin density and T2-weighted images are used to generate Parzen map (*3*) for classifying tissues as white matter (*pink*) or gray matter (*gray*). The composite segmented image (*4*) is formed by hierarchical assignment of BOD1, BOD2, CSF, and gray and white matter based on this nonparametric Parzen window technique. Last, the automatically segmented composite images are reviewed by an experienced operator who eliminates any false lesion classifications due to coherent or noncoherent flow artifacts or excessive patient motion to create the final segmented image (*5*)

were then used to segment all patient images acquired across the study. The segmentation strategy now includes an expert step to remove false lesion identification due to coherent and noncoherent flow artifacts. This step eliminated the need for baseline 3D phase-contrast flow images and the automated removal of residual flow artifacts that occasionally excluded true lesions.

Another potential advantage of the new analysis system is that it adds an additional classification of lesions based on their apparent extent of tissue disruption. Some lesions noted on fluid attenuation by inverse recovery (FLAIR) have low rather than high signal characteristics. As previously noted by others, such lesions in general correspond to hypointense lesions seen on T1-weighted images [20]. These lesions can potentially lead to an underestimation of the total plaque burden seen on FLAIR compared to that found on more conventional T2-weighted images in some cases [21], depending upon the methods used for lesion quantitation. However, the multispectral technique allows an estimate of the fraction of lesions showing increased amounts of loss of tissue integrity using a lesion set that is registered in an absolute sense by the method of image acquisition.

An example of such "textured" tissue destruction within an individual lesion is shown in Fig. 3. In this specific lesion four levels of tissue destruction may be

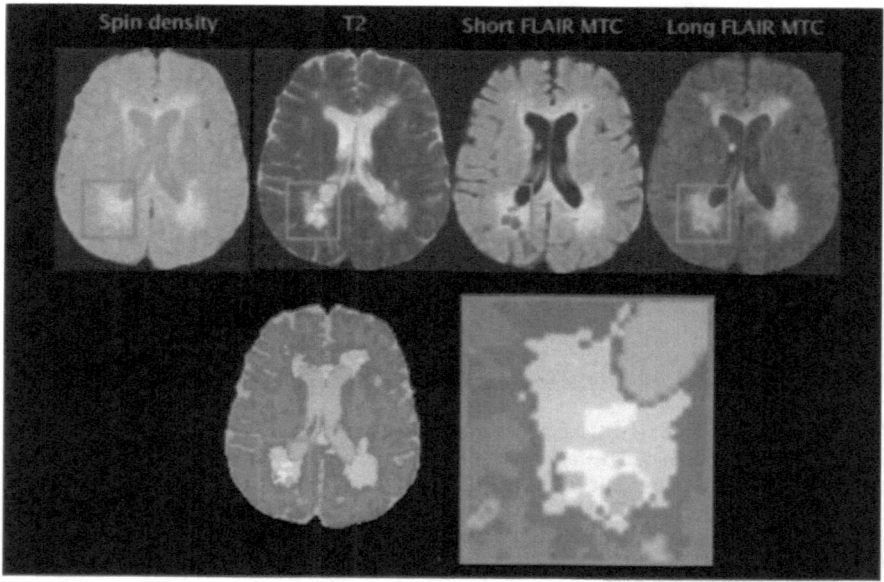

Fig. 3. Extreme tissue heterogeneity is apparent within one of several regions containing MS plaque. The four images of a single 3-mm transaxial tissue slice obtained with the AFFIRMATIVE pulse sequence are displayed in the *top row* of images in this figure for comparison with the final corrected segmented image. The *green box* outlines the area of significant plaque heterogeneity as determined by automated sequence analysis and the detail of the region illustrated in the *lower righthand component* of the composite illustration. Color-coding of the segmented tissues is as described for Fig. 2

noted. The outermost region has been segmented as if it were gray matter even though it is anatomically positioned within white matter. This region of the lesion, depending upon the method of lesion quantitation used, could either be considered as part of the lesion or, more likely, defined as "normal-appearing white matter" or so-called "dirty" white matter. Most quantitation techniques would base this decision on a subjective evaluation of a T2-weighted image. In the automated system, the judgment is based on signal characteristics of an individual voxel using a cross-comparison to four different types of images obtained in a single acquisition with reference to three separate probabilistic maps. The outer edges of the next zone of the lesion generally correspond to the visual extent of the lesions seen on the long echo FLAIR with magnetization transfer contrast (MTC) acquisition (referred to as BOD1). Within this zone of the lesion are two regions corresponding to increasingly severe tissue destruction. The first of these (referred to as BOD2) reflects tissue that is more severely disturbed than that classified as BOD1, but not so severely affected as that classified by the segmentation algorithm as CSF.

In order to obtain some appreciation of the differences and similarities between the old and new segmentation strategies, image analysis was performed using both methods on images obtained from 299 subjects with PPMS. The extent of correlation between these two approaches for the major MRI metrics is displayed in Fig. 4. No change was made in the determination of the extent of

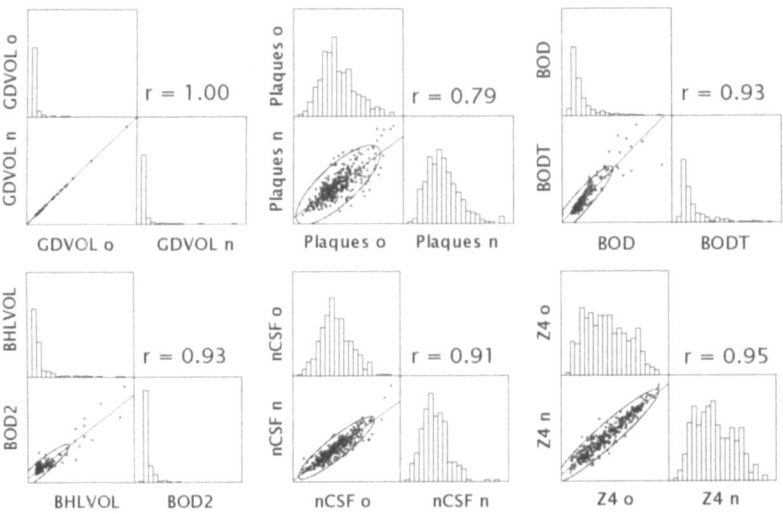

Fig. 4. A series of bivariate scatterplots for each specified pair of variables is displayed for selected MRI metrics determined using the old (*o*) or new (*n*) segmentation strategy. The plots compare enhanced tissue volumes (*GDVOL*), number of discrete plaques (*Plaques*), disease burden as determined by the old (*BOD*) and new (*BODT*) methods, T1-hypointense lesion volume (*BHLVOL*) and new BOD2 from the AFFIRMATIVE images, cerebrospinal fluid as a proportion of the total segmented intracranial contents (*nCSF*), and old and new composite scores (*Z4*). Each scatterplot shows a linear regression line that best fits the data and a sample ellipse that envelopes 95% confidence on the means

gadolinium-enhanced tissues, and this is reflected in the upper left panel of this figure, where there is complete concordance between the two data sets. The number of individual lesions counted showed the least correlation, with an r value of only 0.79. This is not unexpected, given the considerable changes in correcting for false lesion classification. In contrast, the correlation between hypointense lesion volumes obtained on postgadolinium T1-weighted images by manual seeding and those obtained with the new automated image analysis system is in part consistent with the previous observations of others [20]. However, it also is probably a partial reflection of the relatively low enhancement frequency within this patient population, and the fact that our previous strategy excluded portions of hypointense T1-defined lesions whose signal intensity was similar to that of CSF [16].

Our previous estimate of disease burden as defined by AFFIRMATIVE images (BOD) also encompassed tissue that was separately segmented as hypointense lesions on T1-weighted images. Therefore, it is most appropriate to determine the correlation between the old BOD and the new BODT (the sum of the new BOD1 and BOD2). BOD and BODT were highly correlated. Similarly, there was good correlation between the old and new methods of segmenting CSF volume and the proportion of CSF that contributed to all segmented intracranial contents. The change in segmentation methodology dictated a new construct for the Z4 composite. Previously Z4 was defined as an unweighted sum of the Z transformation of the rank values of the enhanced tissue volume, the BOD, the T1 hypointense lesion volume, and the proportion of CSF contributing to the segmented intracranial contents [17]. The new Z4 composite replaces BOD with BODT and the T1 hypointense lesion volume with BOD1. The old and new Z4 composites provided highly correlated results with a somewhat more normal distribution of the values obtained using the new segmentation strategy (Fig. 4).

Correlations Based on New MRI Metrics

The MRI metrics available for the PPMS subjects at entry into the PROMiSe Trial are given in Table 3. These do not reflect all patients who subsequently entered the trial, but those for whom "clean" information was available at the time of presentation of a "snapshot" of the data for the 53rd Annual Meeting of the American Academy of Neurology. Statistically robust correlations were found between many of the MRI measures and clinical demographics of these subjects ($p < 0.0001$ in all instances unless otherwise stated). Age was inversely related to the volume of enhanced tissue found on entry MRI ($r = -0.23$). This inverse correlation of age and enhancement metrics has now been demonstrated to hold across all MS clinical phenotypes [16, 22]. The volume of enhanced tissue also correlated directly with BOD1 ($r = 0.22$). Increasing numbers of discrete plaques were associated directly with longer times required to perform the nine-hole peg test ($r = 0.31$), fewer correct responses on the PASAT 3 ($r = -0.26$), and larger CSF volumes ($r = 0.39$). Not surprisingly, BOD1 was also associated with performance on

Table 3. MRI metrics at entry

	Mean ± SD	95% CI	Median, Range
Enhancement metrics ($n = 730$)			
% Enhanced scans	14.7	12.1, 17.2	0, 0-1
Number of distinct enhancements	0.37 ± 1.46	0.27, 0.48	0, 0-18
Enhanced tissue volume (μl)	32.1 ± 141	21.8, 42.4	0, 0-1,700
Other Metrics ($n = 534$)			
Distinct plaques	132 ± 62.6	127, 138	123, 19-486
BOD1 (ml)	6.96 ± 8.15	6.26, 7.65	3.99, 0.09-49.8
BOD2 (ml)	1.13 ± 1.66	0.99, 1.27	0.63, 0-17.6
BODT (ml)	8.08 ± 9.26	8.09, 8.88	4.76, 0.22-61.3
CSF (ml)	202 ± 62.0	196, 207	194, 62.2-548
nCSF	14.5 ± 3.88	14.1, 14.8	14.0, 5.4-33.2

CI, confidence interval

the nine-hole peg test ($r = 0.31$) and the PASAT 3 ($r = -0.33$), correlated with CSF as a proportion of the total segmented intracranial contents (nCSF; $r = 0.46$), and correlated quite strongly with BOD2 ($r = 0.70$) and BODT ($r = 0.99$). BOD2 showed a less strong relationship with ambulation index ($r = 0.16, p < 0.002$), the nine-hole peg test ($r = 0.25$), and the PASAT 3 ($r = -0.30$). The nCSF as a measure of atrophy correlated with age ($r = 0.34$), performance on the nine-hole peg test ($r = 0.27$), and the PASAT 3 ($r = -0.27$).

The influence of the patient's disability at entry into the trial [based upon their stratification by EDSS score into the low (3.0-5.0) or high (5.5-6.5) stratum] on differences between the MRI metrics was explored. Patients in the higher EDSS stratum had more atrophy as indicated by higher nCSF values (14.8% versus 14.2%, $p < 0.05$) and worse mean Z4 composites scores (Z4 = 0.249 and - 0.297, $p < 0.05$). The other MRI metrics did not differ significantly between the two EDSS strata. When grouped by enhancement status at entry, those with enhancements had significantly higher mean volumes of BOD1 (10.21 versus 6.23), BOD2 (1.47 versus 1.06), and BODT (11.68 versus 7.28) ($p < 0.001$ in all instances). Perhaps of greatest interest were differences found in the MRI metrics when patients were grouped by CSF status (Tab. 4). The subjects whose CSF was abnormal by virtue of the presence of oligoclonal bands, an elevated IgG index, or an elevated IgG synthetic rate had more enhancements, plaques, and larger plaque volumes of all types. As a group, those with no CSF abnormality had better overall MRI metrics as judged by the Z4 composite score.

Discussion

Altogether 943 patients were recruited into this double-blind, placebo-controlled treatment trial that is focused exclusively on patients with PPMS. It is reasonable to suspect that about 0.5%-1.0% of all eligible patients within the catchment

Table 4. MRI metrics at entry by CSF status

	Positive	Negative	p
Enhancement metrics (n)	574	139	
% Enhanced scans	15.7	10.8	NS
Number of distinct enhancements	0.429	0.151	< 0.05
Enhanced tissue volume (μl)	37	12	NS
Other metrics (n)	411	104	
Distinct plaques	136	119	< 0.01
BOD1 (ml)	7.21	4.75	< 0.05
BOD2 (ml)	1.18	0.82	< 0.01
BODT (ml)	8.39	5.60	< 0.05
CSF (ml)	201	202	NS
nCSF	14.4	14.5	NS
Z4 score	0.022	– 0.590	< 0.01

regions of the 58 contributing centers were entered into this study. Thus it is likely that the description of patients with PPMS at entry into this trial is representative of all patients with this disease across the range of age and disability specified by the entry criteria of the trial. As a group, these patients had similar clinical demographics and MRI characteristics to those described for smaller cohorts of patients with PPMS [2, 10, 23, 24].

Until recently, little attention has been focused on patients with PPMS, and diagnostic criteria appropriate for patients with relapsing disease could not easily accommodate PPMS subjects [13, 25, 26]. Recognizing the difficulties in differential diagnosis that are peculiar to PPMS, European neurologists interested in the problem suggested an algorithm for diagnosis based on clinical presentation, MRI characteristics, and CSF findings [11]. In this schema, the presence or absence of oligoclonal bands is central to the degree of clinical diagnostic certainty. Based on this schema, most patients participating in the PROMiSe Trial would be classified as having definite or at least probable PPMS. More recent recommendations of an international panel on the diagnosis of MS suggest that positive findings on CSF analysis are critical for diagnosis of PPMS [12] and therefore would exclude approximately 20% of subjects participating in the PROMiSe Trial as not having PPMS. Undoubtedly, the level of comfort with the clinical diagnosis of PPMS is greatly enhanced by finding CSF abnormalities typical of MS, but others report a similar proportion of patients with negative CSF findings among their PPMS cohort [10]. Further, it is well recognized that even in relapsing forms of MS, CSF evaluation may be normal, particularly in early phases of the disease. In this study, all patients with negative CSF findings had supporting documents reviewed by one or more members of a central patient eligibility review committee to assure that the clinical course was consistent with PPMS, that other competing diagnoses were actively excluded, and that there was other paraclinical evidence to support to the diagnosis (characteristic findings on cerebral or spinal MRI, or abnormalities on visual evoked responses). The longitudinal course of patients entered into studies such as the PROMiSe Trial should provide critical evidence on which to base whether the international recommendations need revision for the diagnosis of PPMS.

Assuming that patients in this study cohort reasonably reflect all patients with PPMS, it is useful to note that these patients have substantially less MRI-defined pathology than comparably clinically impaired patients with either secondary progressive or relapsing-remitting MS. It is also of interest that those patients with positive CSF findings have evidence of more significant plaque burdens on their entry cerebral MRI. Positive CSF findings imply a significant intrathecal production of immunoglobulins, presumably related to infiltration of the central nervous system with B cells. This leads to the possibility that CSF-positive patients with PPMS have a more tissue-destructive disease process than those whose CSF lacks evidence of a B-cell immunopathogenic component to their disease.

Sample size projections for this trial suggest that studies in PPMS must involve reasonably large numbers of patients followed for extended intervals in order to detect with confidence a substantial effect of a drug in slowing progression of clinical impairment. Other studies, either recently completed or ongoing in patients with PPMS (interferon-β1a, interferon-β1b, mitoxantrone, riluzole) have enrolled substantially smaller patient cohorts. If our sample size projections are correct, the smaller studies may face type 2 errors if their outcomes prove negative.

Acknowledgements. This work was supported by a grant from Teva Neuroscience.

Appendix

The PROMiSe Trial Study Group principal investigators, centers, and cities are:

Canada: Lorne Kastrukoff, University of British Columbia, Vancouver; Pierre Duquette, Hôpital Notre Dame, Montreal; Mark Freedman, University of Ottawa Medical Associates, Ottawa; Paul O'Connor, St. Michael's Hospital, Toronto

France: Marc Debouverie, Hôpital Central, Nancy; Catherine Lubetzki, Hopital la Pitié - Salpêtrière, Paris; Gilles Edan, Hôpital Pontchaillou, Rennes; Etienne Roullet, Hôpital Tenon, Paris; Christian Confavreux, Hôpital Neurologique, Lyon

United Kingdom: Alan Thompson, Institute of Neurology, London; Lance Blumhardt, Queens Medical Centre, Nottingham; Stanley Hawkins, Royal Victoria Hospital, Belfast

United States: Thomas Scott, Allegheny General Hospital, Pittsburgh; Daniel Wynn, Consultants in Neurology, Chicago; Joanna Cooper, East Bay Neurology, Berkeley; Stephen Thurston, Henrico Doctor's Hospital, Richmond; Stanton Elias, Henry Ford Hospital, Detroit; Clyde Markowitz, Hospital of the University of Pennsylvania, Philadelphia; David Mattson, Indiana University School of Medicine, Indianapolis; Aaron Miller, Maimonides Medical Center, Brooklyn; John Noseworthy, Mayo Clinic, Rochester; Elizabeth Shuster, Mayo Clinic of Jacksonville, Jacksonville; Jonathan Carter, Mayo Clinic Scottsdale, Scottsdale; Fred Lublin, Medical College of Pennsylvania-Hahneman School of Medicine, Philadelphia; William Stuart, MS Center at Shepherd Center, Atlanta; Michael Kaufman, MS Center of the Carolinas, Charlotte; Gary Birnbaum, MS Treatment and Research Center, Golden Valley; Kottil Rammohan, Ohio State University School of Medicine, Columbus; Ruth Whitham, Oregon Health Science University, Portland; Cornelia Mihai, Research Foundation of the State University of New York, Syracuse; Steven Greenberg, Roswell Park Cancer Center, Buffalo; Craig Smith, Swedish Medical Center, Seattle; Mark Agius,

University of California Davis Medical Center, Davis; Stan van den Noort, University of California Irvine, Irvine; Lawrence Myers, University of California Los Angeles MS Research, Los Angeles; James Nelson, University of California San Diego, La Jolla; Douglas Goodin, University of California San Francisco, San Francisco; Barry Arnason, University of Chicago, Chicago; John Whitaker, University Hospital, Birmingham; Sharon Lynch, University of Kansas Medical Center, Kansas City; Kenneth Johnson, University of Maryland Hospital, Baltimore; Patricia Coyle, University Medical Center at State University of New York, Stony Brook; Stephen Kamin, University Medical and Dental New Jersey Medical School, Newark; William Sheremata, University of Miami School of Medicine, Miami; Corey Ford, University of New Mexico, Albuquerque; Galen Mitchell, University of Pittsburgh MS Center, Pittsburgh; Andrew Goodman, University of Rochester Medical Center, Rochester; Norman Kachuck, University of Southern California, Los Angeles; Peter Dunne, University of South Florida, Tampa; J. William Lindsey, University of Texas Health Science Center, Houston; Elliot Frohman, University of Texas Southwestern Medical Center, Dallas; James Bowen, University of Washington School of Medicine, Seattle; Benjamin Brooks, University of Wisconsin, Madison; John Rose, University of Utah, Salt Lake; Harold Moses, Vanderbilt Stallwort Rehabilitation Center, Nashville; Douglas Jeffrey, Wake Forest University Baptist Medical Center, Winston-Salem; John Trotter, Washington University, St. Louis; Robert Lisak, Wayne State University School of Medicine, Detroit; Tim Vollmer, Yale University School of Medicine, New Haven

Data Safety Monitoring Board: Henry McFarland, chair, Jack Antel, Gary Cutter, Luanne Metz, Stephen Reingold

Teva Neuroscience and Teva Pharmaceuticals, Ltd.: Lillian Pardo, Rob Elfont, Rivka Kreitman, Shaul Kadosh, Galia Shifroni, Irit Pinchasi, Yafit Stark, David Ladkani

MRI Analysis Center: Irina Vainrub, Lucie Lambert, Rimma Boykin, Saria Momin, Fengwei Zhong

References

1. Lublin FD, Reingold SC (1996) Defining the clinical course of multiple sclerosis: results of an international survey. National Multiple Sclerosis Society (USA) Advisory Committee on Clinical Trials of New Agents in Multiple Sclerosis. Neurology 46:907-911
2. Stevenson VL, Miller DH, Rovaris M et al (1999) Primary and transitional progressive MS: a clinical and MRI cross-sectional study. Neurology 52:839-845
3. Poser CM, Paty DW, Scheinberg L et al (1983) New diagnostic criteria for multiple sclerosis: guidelines for research protocols. Ann Neurol 13:227-231
4. European Study Group on interferon beta-1b in secondary progressive MS (1998) Placebo-controlled multicentre randomised trial of interferon beta-1b in treatment of secondary progressive multiple sclerosis. Lancet 352:1491-1497
5. Secondary Progressive Efficacy Clinical Trial of Recombinant Interferon-beta-1a in MS (SPECTRIMS) Study Group (2001) Randomized controlled trial of interferon-beta-1a in secondary progressive MS: Clinical results. Neurology 56:1496-1504
6. Kurtzke JF (1983) Rating neurologic impairment in multiple sclerosis: an expanded disability status scale (EDSS). Neurology 33:1444-1452
7. Weinshenker BG, Bass B, Rice GP et al (1989) The natural history of multiple sclerosis: a geographically based study. I. Clinical course and disability. Brain 112:133-146
8. Cottrell DA, Kremenchutzky M, Rice GP et al (1999) The natural history of multiple sclerosis: a geographically based study. 6. Applications to planning and interpretation of clinical therapeutic trials in primary progressive multiple sclerosis. Brain 122:641-647
9. Bornstein MB, Miller A, Slagle S et al (1991) A placebo-controlled, double-blind, randomized, two-center, pilot trial of Cop 1 in chronic progressive multiple sclerosis.

Neurology 41:533-539
10. McDonnell GV, Hawkins SA (1998) Clinical study of primary progressive multiple sclerosis in Northern Ireland, UK. J Neurol Neurosurg Psychiatry 64:451-6454
11. Thompson AJ, Montalban X, Barkhof F et al (2000) Diagnostic criteria for primary progressive multiple sclerosis: a position paper. Ann Neurol 47:831-835
12. McDonald WI, Compston A, Edan G et al (2001) Recommended diagnostic criteria for multiple sclerosis: Guidelines from the International Panel on the Diagnosis of Multiple Sclerosis. Ann Neurol 50:121-127
13. Thompson AJ, Polman CH, Miller DH et al (1997) Primary progressive multiple sclerosis. Brain 120:1085-1096
14. Cottrell DA, Kremenchutzky M, Rice GP et al (1999) The natural history of multiple sclerosis: a geographically based study. 5. The clinical features and natural history of primary progressive multiple sclerosis. Brain 122:625-639
15. Bedell BJ, Narayana PA, Wolinsky JS (1997) A dual approach for minimizing false lesion classifications on magnetic resonance images. Magn Reson Med 37:94-102
16. Wolinsky JS, Narayana PA, Noseworthy JH et al (2000) Linomide in relapsing and secondary progressive MS: part II: MRI results. MRI Analysis Center of the University of Texas-Houston, Health Science Center, and the North American Linomide Investigators. Neurology 54:1734-1741
17. Wolinsky JS, Narayana PA, Johnson KP, and the Copolymer 1 Multiple Sclerosis Study Group and the MRI Analysis Center (2001) United States open-label glatiramer acetate extension trial for relapsing multiple sclerosis: MRI and clinical correlates. Mult Scler 7:33-41
18. Noseworthy JH, Wolinsky JS, Lublin FD et al (2000) Linomide in relapsing and secondary progressive MS: part I: trial design and clinical results. North American Linomide Investigators. Neurology 54:1726-1733
19. Filippi M, Rovaris M, Gasperini C et al (1998) A preliminary study comparing the sensitivity of serial monthly enhanced MRI after standard and triple dose gadolinium-DTPA for monitoring disease activity in primary progressive multiple sclerosis. J Neuroimaging 8:88-93
20. Rovaris M, Comi G, Rocca MA et al (1999) Relevance of hypointense lesions on fast fluid-attenuated inversion recovery MR images as a marker of disease severity in cases of multiple sclerosis. Am J Neuroradiol 20:813-820
21. van Waesberghe JH, Castelijns JA, Weerts JG et al (1996) Disappearance of multiple sclerosis lesions with severely prolonged T1 on images obtained by a FLAIR pulse sequence. Magn Reson Imaging 14:209-213
22. Filippi M, Wolinsky JS, Sormani MP, Comi G, European Canadian Glatiramer Acetate Study Group (2001) Enhancement frequency decreases with increasing age in relapsing-remitting multiple sclerosis. Neurology 56:422-423
23. Andersson PB, Waubant E, Gee L, Goodkin DE (1999) Multiple sclerosis that is progressive from the time of onset: clinical characteristics and progression of disability. Arch Neurol 56:1138-1142
24. Bashir K, Whitaker JN (1999) Clinical and laboratory features of primary progressive and secondary progressive MS. Neurology 53:765-771
25. McDonnell GV, Hawkins SA (1996) Primary progressive multiple sclerosis: a distinct syndrome? Mult Scler 2:137-141
26. Leary SM, Stevenson VL, Miller DH, Thompson AJ (1999) Problems in designing and recruiting to therapeutic trials in primary progressive multiple sclerosis. J Neurol 246:562-568

Chapter 7

Conventional MRI

G.T. INGLE, A.J. THOMPSON, D.H. MILLER

Introduction

Conventional magnetic resonance (MR) images are obtained from the ^{1}H nuclei in water and fat. The resolution of such images is usually 1 mm × 1 mm in plane with a slice thickness of either 3 or 5 mm. Different tissues can be distinguished by the difference in the density and macromolecular environment of their mobile protons. The intensity of tissue signals is influenced by three main parameters: proton density (PD), T1 relaxation time and T2 relaxation time. T1 and T2 relaxation times define the rate at which the nuclear MR signals decay after the radiofrequency excitation pulse ceases (T1: longitudinal relaxation i.e. parallel to the magnetic field; T2: transverse relaxation, i.e. perpendicular to the magnetic field). PD and T2-weighted spin echo sequences (or their more rapidly acquired modification, the fast spin echo) are the most widely used for diagnostic studies in multiple sclerosis (MS). They have high specificity for tissue abnormality and the relation between MRI and tissue abnormalities in MS has been studied using post-mortem material [1-3].

The typical white matter lesions found macroscopically at post mortem in MS appear on T2-weighted images as areas of clearly demarcated very high signal. Smaller abnormalities on MR images are sometimes difficult to identify macroscopically. At a microscopic level, lesions can show a variety of histological appearances including complete demyelination, remyelination, inflammation, gliosis and variable axonal loss.

When images are acquired with T1 weighting the majority of MS lesions appear as isointense with normal white matter. Some lesions, however, appear hypointense, and this is interpreted as reflecting a loss of tissue structure and an expanded extracellular space. Persistent T1 hypointensity in this context may be a marker of axonal loss [3].

Chelated gadolinium (gadolinium diethyletriaminepentaacetic acid, Gd-DTPA) has a strong paramagnetic effect and shortens the T1 relaxation rate. It is an extracellular contrast agent and is not able to cross the intact blood-brain barrier. Gadolinium enhancement thus is a marker of blood-brain barrier breakdown and histologically correlates with the inflammatory phase of lesion development [4-7].

A summary table of MRI parameters, their detectable physical alterations and their conventional interpretation is given in Table 1.

Table 1. Conventional MRI parameters and their interpretation

MRI parameter	Physical alteration	Interpretation
Gadolinium enhancement	Uptake in central nervous system	Blood-brain barrier disruption
T1 relaxation rate	Mild prolongation	Intracellular oedema, gliosis
	Strong prolongation	Extracellular oedema and axonal loss
T2 relaxation rate	Reduced short component	Loss of myelin-associated water
	Increased long component	Increased free (extracellular) water

It is generally accepted that patients with a primary progressive (PP) clinical history have some distinctive features on conventional MRI. These features can be summarised as follows:

- A relatively low T2 and T1 hypointense lesion load in comparison with other MS subtypes
- A relatively low level of gadolinium enhancement
- A higher rate of diffuse but subtle abnormality.

As for MS more generally, the correlation between conventional MR metrics and clinical measures of disability is weak, but it has been suggested that there may be a greater correlation with measures of atrophy, especially of the spinal cord, in comparison to other subtypes. This chapter will briefly review conventional MR findings by looking first at the initial MRI observations of patients with PPMS and then considering the more detailed studies that have followed in recent years.

Initial Observations

The first study to specifically examine the MRI appearances of PPMS was that of Thompson et al. in 1990 [8]. Thirteen patients with PPMS were studied together with 16 with secondary progressive MS (SPMS) and 12 with benign disease. T2- and T1-weighted images were assessed by two blinded observers. Patients with PPMS had few lesions (the lowest lesion load of all three groups studied, see Tables 2 and 3), and those lesions that were present were small, 85% being under 5 mm in size. By comparison, in SPMS lesions tended to be large and confluent. Distribution of lesions did not differ between the groups in the internal capsule, brain stem and cerebellum, although there was a tendency for patients with PPMS to have fewer lesions in the periventricular area (Table 2). Cortical atrophy (qualitatively assessed) was seen in one patient with PPMS in comparison with one with benign disease and five with SPMS. In this early study spinal cord abnormalities were seen in 3 of 9 patients with PPMS compared to 7 of 16 patients with SPMS and 5 of 11 patients with a benign history.

Table 2. Lesion distribution in primary and secondary progressive multiple sclerosis compared. (from [8])

	PPMS	SPMS	Level of significance
Periventricular	19.2	34.9	$p = 0.003$
Discrete cerebral	15.6	22.0	$p = 0.01$
Internal capsule	1.5	1.9	$p = 0.29$
Brainstem	3.6	3.5	$p = 0.74$
Cerebellum	1.0	1.9	$p = 0.21$
Total	39.4	62.3	

Cerebral T2 and T1 Lesion Loads

Subsequent studies have examined larger populations of patients with PPMS and have quantified lesions on T1- or PD/T2-weighted scans using computer-assisted visual or semi-automated algorithms. Quantitative T2 and T1 lesion load data in PPMS is presented in several studies and these are summarised in Tables 3 and 4 [9-15].

Differences in lesion distribution between PPMS and other subtypes were seen by Filippi et al. in 1995 [9]. Patients with PPMS had lower overall lesion loads than

Table 3. Lesion load visible on T2-weighted MRI in primary progressive multiple sclerosis

Study	Year	RRMS	SPMS	PPMS
Thompson et al. [8]	1990	–	69.0 cm³	38.5 cm³
Thompson et al. [18]	1991	–	62.0 cm³	39.0 cm³
Filippi et al. [9]	1995	–	110.0 cm³	9.0 cm³
Lycklama à Nijeholt et al. [11]	1999	4.1 cm³	11.0 cm³	3.2 cm³
Stevenson et al. [12]	1999	–	27.7 cm³	12.0 cm³
Filippi et al. [13]	1999	14.1 cm³	23.9 cm³	4.3 cm³
Foong et al. [14]	2000	–	39.8 cm³	10.7 cm³
Van Walderveen et al. [15]	2001	4.7 cm³	11.7 cm³	3.6 cm³
Wolinsky (European Neurological Society poster 2001)	2001	15.4 cm³	16.5 cm³	15.6 cm³

Table 4. Lesion load visible on T1-weighted MRI in relapsing-remitting, secondary progressive and primary progressive multiple sclerosis

Study	Year	RRMS	SPMS	PPMS
Lycklama à Nijeholt et al. [11]	1998	0.3 cm³	2.0 cm³	0.3 cm³
Stevenson et al. [12]	1999	–	7.0 cm³	4.3 cm³
Filippi et al. [13]	1999	0.9 cm³	4.9 cm³	0.1 cm³
Van Walderveen et al. [15]	2001	0.3 cm³	2.0 cm³	0.3 cm³
Wolinsky (European Neurological Society poster 2001)	2001	0.5 cm³	1.0 cm³	0.8 cm³

SPMS especially in frontal, occipital horn and trigonal areas and in the parietal and temporal lobes. In this study patients with PPMS manifesting as a progressive spinal cord syndrome had significantly lower cerebral lesion loads than those with clinical evidence of brain involvement.

Lycklama à Nijeholt el al. studied lesion load in both brain and spinal cord of PPMS, SPMS and relapsing-remitting MS (RRMS) [11]. PP patients had fewer cerebral T2 and T1 lesions than SP patients and overall loads were similar to those of an RR group. The ratio of T1 load to T2 load was also found to be less in the PP group. PP patients were, however, found to have a higher incidence of diffuse hyperintense brain abnormalities on PD-weighted images than SP patients (9 of 31 patients against 3 of 28 patients). These diffuse abnormalities were found mostly in the parietal periventricular white matter. An example of similar changes in a patient with PPMS is shown in Fig. 1.

In this study no brain MRI parameter correlated with the Expanded Disability Status Scale (EDSS) score in PPMS. This contrasted with the SP and RR group where there was a correlation between EDSS and all brain parameters.

Further information about the nature of T1 abnormalities in PPMS has been provided by van Walderveen et al. [15]. The T2 and T1 loads of 42 patients with PPMS were compared with those of 52 patients with RRMS and 44 patients with SPMS. In this study the T1 to T2 ratio was only marginally lower in the PP group than in the SP group (ratios of 0.15 and 0.16 respectively). The T1 to T2 ratio in the RR group in this study was 0.07. For PP patients a trend was noted towards higher T1 lesion volumes and a higher T1 to T2 ratio for male patients than for

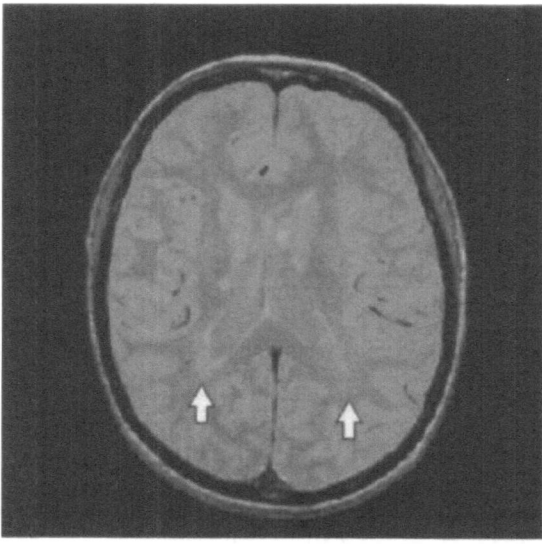

Fig. 1. Areas of diffuse white matter change on a PD-weighted image in a patient with primary progressive multiple sclerosis

female patients. There was no difference either in this group between low and high EDSS score and T1 lesion load, but a trend towards lower T1 lesion volumes and T1 to T2 ratios was noted in patients aged less than 39 years at the onset of symptoms. No such trend was seen for T2 lesion load. Neither T1 or T2 lesion volume correlated with any clinical parameter in the PP group, although associations with T1 lesion volume and EDSS score and disease duration were seen for the RR and SP groups.

The relation of brain lesion load to clinical measures was studied in more detail by Stevenson et al. in a multicentre (six sites) European study [12]. Again, PP patients were seen to have lower mean T2 and T1 lesion loads than SP patients, but in this study, in contrast to those of Lycklama à Nijeholt and Filippi et al. [11, 13], no difference was seen in the T1 to T2 ratio. A trend towards higher T1 lesion load in male than in female PP subjects was also seen at baseline (0.5-0.4 cm^3, $p = 0.04$, unpublished observation). Within the PP group no correlation was found with either EDSS or disease duration. However, both T2 and T1 lesion load correlated with the nine-hole peg test. Interestingly, in a separate analysis of this data reported by Camp et al. [16], a correlation was seen between the cognitive impairment index and both T2 and T1 lesion load. As in the study of Filippi et al. [9], patients with PPMS presenting with a spinal cord syndrome had significantly lower brain T2 and T1 lesion loads. This study also noted a difference in PPMS brain T2 lesion load between study sites despite similar patient ages, disease duration and EDSS.

Change in lesion number and load over time has also been studied. In the study of Stevenson et al. 43.6% of patients with PPMS demonstrated one or more new brain lesions over a 1-year period [17]. Over the same period T2 lesion load increased by a median of 7.3% and T1 lesion load increased by a median of 12.6%. None of the baseline clinical measures were predictive of clinical outcome at 1 year. Despite this, some weak relations have emerged between baseline clinical measures and changes in MRI measures. For example, there was a correlation between baseline EDSS and percentage change in T2 and T1 load over 1 year. When this study was extended to 2 years of follow-up, no additional correlations were found between absolute or percentage change in clinical outcomes and MRI measures. Patients with a cord presentation had lower brain T2 and T1 lesion loads at 2 years and also had a lower median increase in T2 load (personal observations). This study is currently being extended to 5 years in order to provide longer-term information about the dynamics of T2 and T1 lesion load increase.

Gadolinium Enhancement: Single and Triple Dose

Single Dose

Gadolinium enhancement in PPMS was first studied by Thompson et al. in 1991 [18]. A group of 24 patients with PPMS and SPMS matched for age, disease duration and disability (12 in each group) were examined over a 6-month period. Scans were carried out every 2 weeks for 3 months and then monthly. On each occasion Gd-DTPA was injected at a dose of 0.1mmol/kg. Of 129 new lesions seen over the 6-month period, 109 were in 11 of 12 SPMS patients, while only 20 new lesions were seen in 6 of 12 patients with PPMS. The rate of development of new lesions was 3.3 lesions per patient per year in the PP group and 18.2 lesions per patient per year in the SP group. Of the 109 new lesions seen in the SP group, 91 showed enhancement with Gd-DTPA, compared to only 1 of 20 new lesions seen in the PP group.

A further serial study examining brain and cord in 10 PP and 9 SP patients was carried out by Kidd et al. in 1996 [19]. Monthly MRI of the brain and spinal cord was carried out with and without gadolinium enhancement over a period of 1 year. MRI activity was again seen to be low in patients with PPMS, with only 20 and 112 lesions in the PP and SP groups respectively.

Early data from a very large cohort of patients (943) with PPMS participating in the international clinical trial of glatiramer acetate have recently been presented (Wolinsky, European Neurological Society poster 2001; see also Chap. 7, this volume). Baseline MR images of 541 patients with PPMS were compared with identically processed baseline images from 92 patients with RRMS and 626 patients with SPMS who had participated in a separate trial. A striking finding was the very low mean volume of gadolinium-enhancing lesions (single dose): this was 0.03 ml on average in PPMS, compared with 0.4 ml in the RR group and 0.2 ml in the SP group.

Triple Dose

The effects of triple-dose Gd-DTPA in PPMS were studied by Filippi et al. in 1995 [20]. Ten patients were examined over two sessions. In the first session, patients were scanned 5-7 min after the injection of 0.1 mmol/kg Gd-DTPA (standard dose). In the second session, 6-24 hours later, patients were scanned once before and twice after the injection of 0.3 mmol/kg Gd-DTPA (triple dose). The post Gd-DTPA scans were carried out at 5-7 min and 1-h after injection. Four enhancing lesions were detected in two patients when the standard dose of Gd-DTPA was used. The numbers of enhancing lesions increased to 13 and the numbers of patients with such lesions to 5 when the triple dose of Gd-DTPA was used, and again to 14 lesions and 6 patients in the 1-h delayed scans. The mean contrast ratio for enhancing lesions detected with the triple dose of Gd-DTPA was higher than those for both the standard dose and the 1-h delayed scans.

The use of triple-dose gadolinium and delayed imaging in PPMS was also examined by Silver et al. in 1997 [21]. Fifty patients were studied including 16 with PPMS. Imaging was performed on two occasions with single- and triple-dose Gd-DTPA. Patients were imaged within early (0-20 min), short-delay (20-40 min) and long-delay (40-60 min) time windows. Whereas triple dose and delay increased the yield of enhancing lesions in the RR and SP groups, there was no such increase in PP patients. Quantitative signal changes were measured in seven PP patients to evaluate non-enhancing lesions and there was a significant signal increase in non-enhancing lesions, suggesting that low-grade blood-brain barrier leakage exists. There was a trend to increased signal in normal-appearing white matter, raising the possibility of an even more diffuse blod-brain barrier abnormality [22]. However, more sensitive methods will be needed to definitively study this issue.

An unresolved issue is whether there may be an early inflammatory phase in PPMS. Since it can take some time for the diagnosis of PPMS to become established, patients included in MRI studies have tended to have established disease, with a disease duration usually over 5 years and often considerably more. A recent preliminary study of patients with disease duration of less than 5 years has shown a higher degree of enhancement (present in 11 of 20 patients initially studied). An example of an enhancing lesion in a patient with PPMS and a disease duration of 3 years is shown in Fig. 2.

Normal-Appearing Tissue: Additional Studies Using Conventional MRI to Measure T1 and T2 Relaxation

By definition normal-appearing white matter is normal in terms of its appearance on conventional MRI, and the identification of its subtle abnormalities has largely awaited the development of so-called non-conventional MRI methods such as magnetisation transfer imaging, diffusion tensor imaging and magnetic resonance spectroscopy (discussed in detail in other chapters of this book). In an early study, however, Thompson et al. showed that T1 relaxation times in an area of frontal normal-appearing white matter were higher in SPMS than in PPMS subjects, whose values were higher than, but not significantly different from,

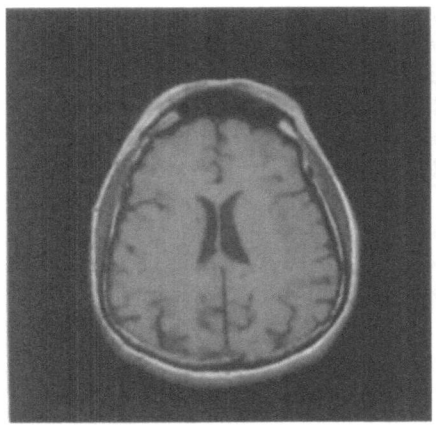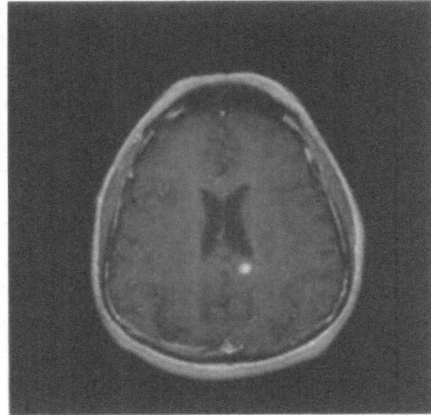

a   b

Fig. 2. T1-weighted images in a patient with primary progressive multiple sclerosis before (*a*) and after (*b*) injection of triple-dose Gd-DTPA

those of control subjects [8]. A relationship was found between T1 values and lesion load. T2 relaxation times were similar in all groups.

Cord

Patients with PPMS often have prominent spinal cord symptoms, and one possible explanation for the disparity of low levels of brain abnormality despite significant disability would be that there is a correspondingly greater degree of abnormality in the spinal cord. Kidd et al. observed that patients with PPMS have a slightly greater percentage of total load due to cord lesions than patients with SPMS (11.8% versus 8.2%) [23]. For some patients with PPMS, conventional MRI abnormalities may be entirely confined to the cord. An example of a cervical cord lesion is shown in Fig. 3. Thorpe studied 11 patients with PPMS with normal or near-normal brain MRI appearances [24]. All patients had at least one lesion visible in the spinal cord. Despite this, an entirely normal conventional brain MRI examination in PPMS is unusual and in one retrospective study was estimated to be found in less than 5% of cases [25].

A requirement for MRI abnormalities to be present in either brain or cord has been incorporated into recently published diagnostic criteria for PPMS [26]. Given that spinal cord lesions are more specific than brain lesions and do not occur with aging [24], the presence of only two discrete spinal cord lesions is regarded as positive MRI evidence according to these criteria even if brain MRI is normal. Nine lesions on brain MRI are otherwise regarded as providing positive MRI evidence, but should one spinal cord lesion be present, only four to eight brain lesions are required.

Lycklama à Nijeholt studied spinal cord appearances in 31 PPMS patients, 28 with RRMS and 32 with SPMS in 1998 [11]. No significant differences were found between clinical subtypes in the number of focal spinal T2 lesions. An interesting observation was that there was an increased likelihood of finding patients with diffuse change within the spinal cord. Diffuse spinal cord abnormalities were seen mainly in SP and PP patients (10 of 32 and 19 of 31 patients, respectively). An example of diffuse change in a patient with PPMS is shown in Fig. 4. In comparison, such abnormalities were present in only 6 out of 28 patients with RRMS. The presence of diffuse spinal cord abnormalities without focal lesions may be an even more specific feature of PP disease. It was seen in 10 of 31 PP patients but in only 4 of 32 SP patients, and was entirely absent in the 28 RR patients.

Conventional MR appearances of the cervical cord were studied by Filippi et al. in 2000 in a study that also examined magnetisation transfer [27]. Nine patients with PPMS were studied together with 41 with RRMS and 31 with SPMS. Abnormal cervical cord scans were found in 81.8% of the PP patients, compared with 78.8% of RR patients and 94% of patients with SPMS. PP patients had a mean of 1.8 cervical cord lesions, while the means for RR and SP patients were 1.7 and 2.5 respectively. The extent of cord damage was reflected by the mean number of cervical cord slices showing lesions: this was 3.2 for the PP group, 4.4

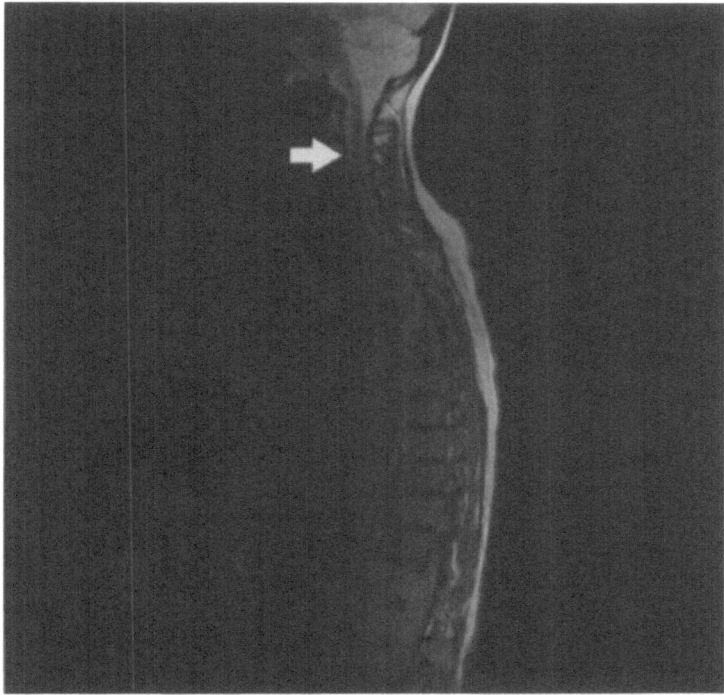

Fig. 3. Area of focal hyperintensity in the cervical cord in a patient with primary progressive multiple sclerosis

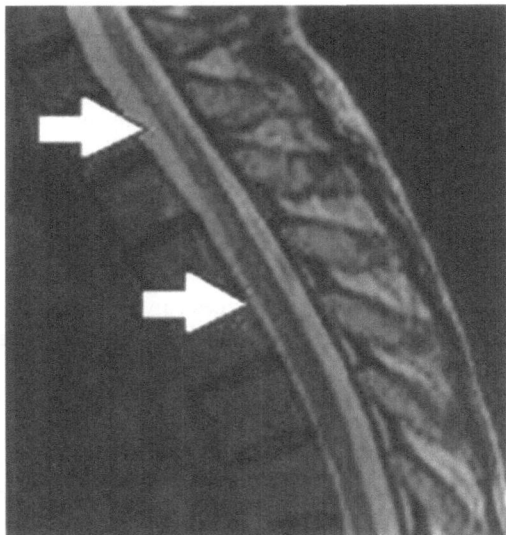

Fig. 4. Areas of diffuse abnormality in the spinal cord of a patient with primary progressive multiple sclerosis

for the SP group and 2.7 for RR patients. SP patients had a higher number of lesions and greater number of slices involved than the other two groups ($p = 0.04$ in each case).

The number of focal spinal lesions in PPMS was also found to be lower than in SPMS in the study of Stevenson et al. [12, 17] (means 1.9 and: 3.2 respectively, $p = 0.04$). At baseline, there was no correlation between spinal cord lesion load and disability. Over 1 year, 25.5% of patients had one or more new cord lesions. Change in EDSS correlated with percentage increase in number and load of spinal cord lesions ($r = 0.19$, $p = 0.005$). No correlation was seen with the number of brain lesions. At baseline, when patients with PPMS with cord presentations were compared with those without, they were not found to differ in terms of lesion load. Over 1 year, the number of new cord lesions was higher in the cord presentation group compared to the non-cord presentation group, but this did not reach significance.

Further information about MRI and histological abnormalities in the spinal cord has recently been provided by a study comparing MRI appearances of the cord at post mortem at two field strengths (4.7 T and 1 T) together with histology. Seven patients with PPMS were included in this study. MRI appearances suggested extensive involvement of the spinal cord, but mainly with a mild signal intensity increase and little involvement of grey matter (in comparison with the cords of patients with SPMS). Interestingly, a greater degree of abnormality was present on MRI than was detected histopathologically. Areas of high signal intensity on MRI corresponded with areas of complete demyelination identified histologically. Areas of mildly increased signal corresponded with areas of partial demyelination.

In summary, PPMS may show abnormalities in the cord when none are detectable in the brain, but there does not necessarily seem to be a particularly high or extensive focal lesion load compared to other MS subtypes. Some correlation may exist between lesion load and disability, and it has been suggested that a greater degree of diffuse abnormality (corresponding histologically to partial demyelination) may be a characteristic feature. Other evidence relating to cord changes in PPMS comes from studies of atrophy measures. These will be considered in the next section.

Atrophy Measures

Conventional MRI sequences can also be used to provide measures of tissue volume and area, which in turn can be used to detect tissue atrophy either by comparing values in a single subject over time or by making comparisons with a control population at a single time point. Atrophy in the central nervous system may be due to changes in grey or white matter or both. Inflammation within tissue may cause a volume increase (due to water and cells) that may prevent atrophy due to tissue loss from being seen. From a limited number of studies performed to date, there is evidence to suggest that global atrophy in PPMS is modest.

Cross-sectional area of the spinal cord at four levels (C5, T2, T7 and T11) was studied by Kidd et al. in patients with PPMS and SPMS over a period of 1 year [19]. A reduction in cord area was seen in both groups that was most pronounced at the C5 level and was greatest in the SP group (a median change of – 5.39 mm^2 compared to a median change of – 2.62 mm^2). When both groups of progressive patients were considered together there was no correlation between change in cord area at any of the four levels and change in EDSS. There was, however, a trend towards a significant difference between change in cord area between those who changed less than 1.0 on EDSS and those whose change was greater (greater change in EDSS being associated with greater change in cord area). This trend was most noticeable at C5.

A larger median spinal cord area in PPMS compared to SPMS was also found by Lycklama à Nijeholt et al. [11]. There was an association between cross-sectional cord area in the PP patients and the number of spinal cord segments showing diffuse involvement. Losseff et al. studied spinal cord area at C2 in 15 patients with PPMS [28]. Their median cord area was 73.1 mm^2, compared to 61.2 mm^2 in SPMS and 85.6 in RRMS and 84.7 mm^2 in controls.

Stevenson et al. studied atrophy measures in both spinal cord and brain [12, 17]. The spinal measure was cervical cord area at the level of C2 using the technique of Losseff et al. [28]. Once again, spinal cord area was smaller in SP patients (64.1-72.7 mm^2), although EDSS was not equal in the two groups studied. Six-slice partial brain volume above the level of the third ventricle was used as a measure of cerebral atrophy [29]. No differences were seen between groups at baseline. Over 1 year measurable changes in both measures were seen in PP patients, with a median change of – 2.3% in partial brain volume and – 2.9% in cord area. There was no correlation with clinical measures, and patients presenting with cord syndromes did not differ in terms of brain or cord atrophy from those presenting in other ways.

Alternative measures of cerebral atrophy are provided by ventricular and cerebrospinal fluid (CSF) volumes. Wolinsky (European Neurological Society poster 2001) studied CSF volume normalised to total segmented intracranial contents. Average CSF volume in PPMS was 15.8 ml, compared to 17.1 ml in RRMS and 17.8 ml in SPMS. Patients with higher EDSS had larger CSF volumes. Ventricular volume was measured on T1-weighted images by Lycklama à Nijeholt et al. [11]. In this study ventricular volume was greatest in SP patients, at 31.9 ml compared to 21.3 ml in PP patients and 22.3 ml in RR disease. In PP patients there was an association between ventricular volume and pyramidal functional systems score.

Conclusions

Later studies have supported the original observations that patients with PPMS develop fewer T2 lesions in the brain, have less T1 hypointensity and have a lower frequency of MRI-detected inflammatory lesions than SP patients despite comparable levels of disability. Conventional MRI studies suggest that there may be less focal inflammatory activity in PPMS in comparison to other subtypes, and there is support for this view from histopathological studies comparing the appearances of PPMS and SPMS [30]. A summary, adapted from Lycklama à Nijeholt et al. [11], is shown in Table 5.

Given that conventional MRI abnormalities are nevertheless present in PPMS, and given that measurable changes in MRI measures can be detected over quite short periods of time, there is a role for MRI monitoring in treatment trials in PPMS as an adjunct to clinical assessment. The poor correlation between conventional MRI measures and disability probably results partly from the poor pathological specificity of these measures and partly from the fact that global measures of disease burden may not always capture important regional differences in lesion load. For example, it is likely that the degree of clinical impairment is dependent on the severity of a few specific lesions located in specific tracts. To date, the approaches adopted for the use of conventional MRI in the monitoring of clinical trials in PPMS have been similar to those used in RRMS and SPMS [31]. Further observation of the natural history, particularly over extended periods, is likely to be helpful in aiding interpretation of treatment effects on conventional MRI measures where these are seen.

Although levels of MRI abnormality are lower in PPMS than other subtypes, an entirely normal conventional MRI appearance is unusual, occurring in an estimated fewer than 5% of cases. This is acknowledged in recently published diagnostic criteria for PPMS [26]. A diagnosis of definite PPMS, according to this consensus statement, requires the presence of nine brain lesions or two spinal lesions or four to eight brain lesions and one spinal lesion.

Administration of Gd-DTPA at either single or triple dose remains an important adjunct to conventional MRI techniques. Lower levels of lesion enhancement in PPMS patients of established diagnosis has been shown in several studies. It is currently less clear whether this is also true for the earliest stages of the condition. Preliminary analysis of a cohort of patients with PPMS and short disease dura-

Table 5. Summary table of conventional MRI features of primary progressive multiple sclerosis. (Adapted from [11])

Measure	RRMS	SPMS	PPMS
Brain			
Focal T2 lesions	Many	Many	Moderate or few
Enhancing lesions	Often	Often	Seldom
Focal T1 lesions	Few	Many	Few
Diffuse abnormalities	Seldom	Variable	Frequent
Ventricular enlargement	Mild	Moderate or marked	Mild
Spine			
Focal T2 lesions	Frequent	Frequent	Frequent
Focal T1 lesions	Never	Never	Never
Diffuse abnormalities	Seldom	Variable	Frequent
Spinal cord atrophy	Mild	Marked	Moderate

tion has shown a higher than expected frequency of enhancing lesions. The finding of subtle quantitative signal alterations after gadolinium injection suggests that low-grade blood-brain barrier leakage may exist in visibly non-enhancing PPMS; it is not clear whether this is pathogenically significant.

In summary, although newer MRI techniques offer the possibility of greater pathological specificity, conventional MR measures will retain their place in the assessment of patients with PPMS for some time to come, both for diagnosis and for monitoring of treatment. Methods of image acquisition and processing continue to improve and the ability to detect subtle changes in tissue volumes (atrophy) seems particularly promising.

References

1. Stewart WA, Hall LD, Berry K, Paty DW (1984) Correlation between NMR scan and brain slice data in multiple sclerosis. Lancet 2:412
2. Newcombe J, Hawkins CP, Henderson CL et al (1991) Histopathology of multiple sclerosis lesions detected by magnetic resonance imaging in unfixed postmortem central nervous system tissue. Brain 114:1013-1023
3. van Waesberghe JH, Kamphorst W, De Groot CJ et al (1999) Axonal loss in multiple sclerosis lesions: magnetic resonance imaging insights into substrates of disability. Ann Neurol 46:747-754
4. Hawkins CP, Munro PM, MacKenzie F et al (1990) Duration and selectivity of blood-brain barrier breakdown in chronic relapsing experimental allergic encephalomyelitis studied by gadolinium-DTPA and protein markers. Brain 113:365-378
5. Katz D, Taubenberger JK, Cannella B et al (1993) Correlation between magnetic resonance imaging findings and lesion development in chronic, active multiple sclerosis. Ann Neurol 34:661-669
6. Nesbit GM, Forbes GS, Scheithauer BW et al (1991) Multiple sclerosis: histopathologic and MR and/or CT correlation in 37 cases at biopsy and three cases at autopsy. Radiology 180:467-474
7. Bruck W, Bitsch A, Kolenda H et al (1997) Inflammatory central nervous system demyelination: correlation of magnetic resonance imaging findings with lesion pathology. Ann Neurol 42:783-793
8. Thompson AJ, Kermode AG, MacManus DG et al (1990) Patterns of disease activity in multiple sclerosis: clinical and magnetic resonance imaging study. Br Med J 300:631-634
9. Filippi M, Campi A, Martinelli V et al (1995) A brain MRI study of different types of chronic-progressive multiple sclerosis. Acta Neurol Scand 91:231-233
10. Gayou A, Brochet B, Dousset V (1997) Transitional progressive multiple sclerosis: a clinical and imaging study. J Neurol Neurosurg Psychiatry 63:396-398
11. Lycklama à Nijeholt GJ, van Walderveen MA, Castelijns JA et al (1998) Brain and spinal cord abnormalities in multiple sclerosis. Correlation between MRI parameters, clinical subtypes and symptoms. Brain 121:687-697
12. Stevenson VL, Miller DH, Rovaris M et al (1999) Primary and transitional progressive MS: a clinical and MRI cross-sectional study. Neurology 52:839-845
13. Filippi M, Iannucci G, Tortorella C et al (1999) Comparison of MS clinical phenotypes using conventional and magnetization transfer MRI. Neurology 52:588-594
14. Foong J, Rozewicz L, Chong WK et al (2000) A comparison of neuropsychological deficits in primary and secondary progressive multiple sclerosis. J Neurol 247:97-101
15. van Walderveen MA, Lycklama ANG, Ader HJ et al (2001) Hypointense lesions on T1-

weighted spin-echo magnetic resonance imaging: relation to clinical characteristics in subgroups of patients with multiple sclerosis. Arch Neurol 58:76-81

16. Camp SJ, Stevenson VL, Thompson AJ et al (1999) Cognitive function in primary progressive and transitional progressive multiple sclerosis: a controlled study with MRI correlates. Brain 122:1341-1348

17. Stevenson VL, Miller DH, Leary SM et al (2000) One year follow up study of primary and transitional progressive multiple sclerosis. J Neurol Neurosurg Psychiatry 68:713-718

18. Thompson AJ, Kermode AG, Wicks D et al (1991) Major differences in the dynamics of primary and secondary progressive multiple sclerosis. Ann Neurol 29:53-62

19. Kidd D, Thorpe JW, Kendall BE et al (1996) MRI dynamics of brain and spinal cord in progressive multiple sclerosis. J Neurol Neurosurg Psychiatry 60:15-19

20. Filippi M, Campi A, Martinelli V et al (1995) Comparison of triple dose versus standard dose gadolinium-DTPA for detection of MRI enhancing lesions in patients with primary progressive multiple sclerosis. J Neurol Neurosurg Psychiatry 59:540-544

21. Silver NC, Good CD, Barker GJ et al (1997) Sensitivity of contrast enhanced MRI in multiple sclerosis. Effects of gadolinium dose, magnetization transfer contrast and delayed imaging. Brain 120:1149-1161

22. Molyneux PD, Kappos L, Polman C et al (2000) The effect of interferon beta-1b treatment on MRI measures of cerebral atrophy in secondary progressive multiple sclerosis Brain 123:2256-2263

23. Kidd D, Thorpe JW, Thompson AJ et al (1993) Spinal cord MRI using multi-array coils and fast spin echo. II. Findings in multiple sclerosis. Neurology 43:2632-2637

24. Thorpe JW, Kidd D, Moseley IF et al (1996) Spinal MRI in patients with suspected multiple sclerosis and negative brain MRI. Brain 119:709-714

25. Kremenchutzky M, Lee D, Rice GP, Ebers GC (2000) Diagnostic brain MRI findings in primary progressive multiple sclerosis. Mult Scler 6:81-85

26. Thompson AJ, Montalban X, Barkhof F et al (2000) Diagnostic criteria for primary progressive multiple sclerosis: a position paper. Ann Neurol 47:831-835

27. Filippi M, Bozzali M, Horsfield MA et al (2000) A conventional and magnetization transfer MRI study of the cervical cord in patients with MS. Neurology 54:207-213

28. Losseff NA, Webb SL, O'Riordan JI, Page R, Wang L et al (1996) Spinal cord atrophy and disability in multiple sclerosis. A new reproducible and sensitive MRI method with potential to monitor disease progression. Brain 119:701-708

29. Losseff NA, Wang L, Lai HM, Yoo DS, Gawne-Cain ML et al (1996) Progressive cerebral atrophy in multiple sclerosis. A serial MRI study. Brain 119:2009-2019

30. Revesz T, Kidd D, Thompson AJ et al (1994) A comparison of the pathology of primary and secondary progressive multiple sclerosis. Brain 117:759-765

31. Leary SM, Stevenson VL, Miller DH, Thompson AJ (1999) Problems in designing and recruiting to therapeutic trials in primary progressive multiple sclerosis. J Neurol 246:562-568

Chapter 8

Magnetization Transfer and Diffusion Tensor Magnetic Resonance Imaging

M. Rovaris, G. Comi, M. Filippi

Introduction

Patients with primary progressive (PP) multiple sclerosis (MS) represent a subgroup with clinical and magnetic resonance (MR) imaging (MRI) characteristics which differ from those of patients with relapsing-remitting (RR) MS or secondary progressive (SP) MS [1, 2]. Although they experience a progressive disease course from onset, the burden and activity of lesions on their T2-weighted and gadolinium-enhanced brain MRI scans are, on average, lower than those seen in other MS phenotypes [3-8]. That the pathology of lesions in PPMS is characterized by a predominant loss of myelin and axons with only mild inflammatory components [9] can explain, at least partially, the relative paucity of conventional MRI-detectable activity [4, 5]. However, unlike the case of other disease phenotypes, in PPMS patients the correlation between MRI abnormalities and clinical disease severity is not significantly ameliorated in relation to the load of brain T1-hypointense lesions [7, 8], which are thought to reflect areas where severe tissue disruption has occurred [10]. Two factors might explain the discrepancy between brain MRI and clinical findings in PPMS: first, the presence of diffuse tissue damage at a microscopic level [11], and, second, a prevalent involvement of the cervical cord [6, 7], which might also explain the disproportion between the severity of locomotor disability and the less pronounced impairment of other functional systems [1].

Magnetization transfer MRI (MT MRI) [12] and diffusion tensor MRI (DT MRI) [13] are neuroimaging techniques that can provide information on the presence and extent of tissue damage with greater pathological specificity than conventional MRI can offer. In addition, they enable us to quantify the severity of tissue pathology affecting the normal-appearing white (NAWM) and gray (NAGM) matter beyond the resolution of conventional MRI. This makes MT and DT MRI promising tools for the study of PPMS, with the potential to provide us with valuable information that will improve our understanding of the pathophysiology of PPMS and to enable us to achieve more accurate monitoring of the evolution of this condition.

MT and DT MRI: Theory and Applications to the Study of MS

MT MRI can provide an index, called the MT ratio (MTR), which reflects the efficiency of the magnetization exchange between protons in tissue water (relatively free) and those bound to the macromolecules [12]. This exchange depends upon the relative concentrations of the two pools of protons and on their efficiency of interaction. Although in MS low MTR values may be caused either by a reduction in the integrity of the macromolecular matrix, reflecting damage to the myelin or to the axonal membrane [14], or by a dilution of the macromolecules brought about by inflammatory edema [14], studies with animal models [15, 16] have shown that MTR reduces only slightly with edema, but more strongly with severe demyelination and axonal loss in lesions of experimental allergic encephalo-myelitis [15] or lysolecithin-induced demyelination [16]. Another study [17], using an animal model of toxic demyelination undergoing spontaneous repair, has shown that MTR recovery is significantly correlated with the occurrence of remyelination. In addition, a postmortem study [18] has provided the most com-pelling evidence that marked reductions of MTR values in MS lesions and NAWM are strongly correlated with the percentage of residual axons and the degree of demyelination.

DT MRI allows quantitative measurements of different aspects of tissue microstructure, obtained by exploiting the properties of water diffusion in the brain [19]. The diffusion coefficient of biological tissues, which is influenced by their various components, including cell membranes and organelles, is always lower than the diffusion coefficient in free water, and for this reason is called the apparent diffusion coefficient (ADC). Pathological processes which modify tissue integrity, resulting in a loss or increased permeability of "restricting" barriers to water molecular motion, can cause an increase in the ADC [20]. Since some cellu-lar structures are aligned on the scale of an image pixel, the measurement of dif-fusion is also dependent on the direction in which diffusion is measured. As a consequence, diffusion measurements can give information about the size, shape, orientation, and geometry of tissues [21]. A measure of diffusion which is inde-pendent of the orientation of structures is provided by the mean diffusivity ($\bar{D}$), the average of the ADCs measured in three orthogonal directions. A full charac-terization of diffusion can be obtained in terms of a tensor [22], a 3×3 matrix which accounts for the correlation existing between molecular displacement along orthogonal directions. From the tensor, it is possible to derive $\bar{D}$, equal to one-third of its trace, and some other dimensionless indices of anisotropy. One of the most used is fractional anisotropy (FA) [23]. Tissue disruption, by removing structural barriers to water molecular motion, typically causes increased $\bar{D}$ and decreased FA values [22, 23]. The pathological elements in MS can alter the per-meability or geometry of structural barriers to water diffusion in the brain. The application of DT MRI to MS is therefore appealing since it can provide quantita-tive estimates of the degree of tissue damage and, as a consequence, might improve our understanding of the mechanisms leading to irreversible disability. Although there are no correlative studies between DT MRI and pathological find-ings, several in vivo DT MRI studies [24-31] have consistently reported increased $\bar{D}$ and decreased FA values in T2-visible lesions and NAWM from MS patients. As expected, the loss of structural barriers is greater in macroscopic lesions, and its magnitude seems to be correlated with the intrinsic tissue damage. Since "inflammatory" changes and gliosis could potentially restrict water molecular motion, myelin and axonal loss are the most likely contributors to DT MRI abnormalities in MS NAWM and lesions.

The analysis of MT MRI and DT MRI scans can be conducted using a region-of-interest (ROI) approach or, on a more global basis, by creating histograms of MTR, $\bar{D}$, or FA values from a given portion of tissue [32, 33]. The latter technique can be applied to the whole of the brain parenchyma, after removal of pixels belonging to cerebrospinal fluid and extracranial tissue. Macroscopic MS lesions segmented on T2-weighted images can also be superimposed onto the coregistered MT MRI or DT MRI scans and the corresponding areas can be masked out, thus obtaining maps and histograms of MTR, $\bar{D}$, or FA from the normal-appearing brain tissue (NABT) in isolation. Another approach is the creation of histograms from the gray and white matter separately, using semi- or fully automated techniques for segmenting these two tissue compartments [34, 35]. MTR histogram analysis has also been applied to the study of the cervical cord and proved to be well correlated to MS-related disability [36].

MT MRI Studies

Brain

The first report of MT MRI findings in PPMS was that from Gass et al. [37], who studied 43 MS patients, ten of whom were affected by PPMS, using a ROI analysis of T2-visible lesions and NAWM. The average lesion MTR was lower in PPMS patients than in subjects with small-vessel disease, but no difference was found between PPMS and other disease phenotypes. A significant inverse correlation between lesion MTR and Expanded Disability Status Scale (EDSS) [38] scores was found for SPMS, but not for PPMS patients. More recently, Leary et al. [39] have used the same analysis method to compare NAWM MTR values from 52 PPMS patients with those from the white matter of healthy controls. The average MTR value from all the ROIs was significantly lower in patients than in controls. When comparing the individual anatomical sites, the difference between PPMS and controls was still significant for the corpus callosum, the centra semiovalia, and the frontal lobe NAWM. A moderate inverse correlation ($r = -0.35$) was found between patients' EDSS and corpus callosum NAWM MTR. Both these studies support the hypothesis that, in PPMS patients, there is diffuse tissue damage in the NAWM, which might contribute, at least partially, to clinical disability.

Two cross-sectional studies [40, 41] have compared brain MTR histogram findings from patients with the major clinical phenotypes of MS, i.e., PP, RR, benign, and SP [42]. Filippi et al. [40] studied ten patients with PPMS and found that among the MS subgroups they had the lowest T2- and T1-visible lesion loads and the highest average lesion MTR, while the MTR histogram peak height was lower than in any other MS phenotype. In this study, formal statistics were based on a priori comparisons, the nature of which was decided on the basis of the patterns of clinical MS evolution. Therefore, findings from PPMS patients were compared with those from healthy controls, and only the MTR histogram peak height was found to be significantly lower in the former than in controls. Interestingly, average brain MTR values were similar in PPMS and benign MS. Dehmeshki et al. [41] performed a similar study in a larger sample (46 cases) of PPMS patients and found no significant differences between PP and RR or SP patients as regards whole-brain MTR histogram-derived quantities. There was no relationship between individual histogram metrics and PPMS patients' EDSS scores, whereas a relationship was found in RR and SP MS. However, when a principal component analysis using all the available histogram data was run, a moderate correlation emerged with PPMS clinical disability ($r = 0.40$).

Since in both these studies [40, 41] the whole of the brain tissue was used to create MTR histograms, it is difficult to disentangle the relative contributions of MS damage occurring within and that occurring outside T2-visible lesions to the observed MTR changes in PPMS, although, given the relative low lesion burden generally observed in these patients, it is conceivable to hypothesize a major contribution from the NABT. This has been confirmed by a preliminary study from Tortorella et al. [43], who obtained MTR histograms of the NABT in isolation. Despite the fact that only ten PPMS patients were studied [43], a significant reduction of all the NABT MTR histogram-derived metrics except for histogram peak position was observed in the comparison with healthy controls, and, similarly to what was found for the whole of the brain tissue [40], histogram peak height was lower in PPMS than in any other MS phenotype. Although a large extent of the NABT is constituted of NAWM and, as a consequence, diffuse NAWM damage is likely to be the major contributor to the observed MTR histogram changes, two preliminary studies have suggested that both NAWM MTR and NAGM MTR are reduced in PPMS patients [35, 44].

A major limitation in interpreting the results of all the above-mentioned studies [35, 40, 41, 43, 44] is the small size of the PPMS patient samples studied, which reflects the low prevalence of this phenotype in the overall MS population [1]. Against this background, we have recently conducted a cross-sectional study [45] in a cohort of 91 PPMS patients, whose conventional MRI and MT MRI findings were compared with those from 30 age-matched healthy controls and 36 SPMS patients with similar levels of disability. The enrollment of such a large sample was made possible by the cooperation between several Italian MS centers, although MRI data acquisition and analysis were always performed in our Institution. In accordance with recently developed diagnostic criteria for PPMS [46], about 85% of our patients were classified as having definite PPMS, indicating that there was careful selection in order to exclude other neurological disorders which have the potential to mimic PPMS clinically. MTR histogram analysis confirmed the presence of diffuse abnormalities in the brain of PPMS patients, for whom the histographic quantities were all significantly lower that those of healthy subjects. The severity of global brain tissue damage was found to be similar in PPMS and SPMS patients. Although PPMS patients showed a significant decrease of brain parenchymal volume with respect to healthy controls, the results of group comparisons for MTR histogram-derived quantities did not change after correcting for this factor, thus indicating that brain atrophy per se causes only minor changes in the characteristics of patients' MTR histograms. Unlike a previous study [43], we did not find brain and NABT MTR histogram differences between PPMS and SPMS patients. This indicates that, in both PPMS and SPMS, progressive reduction of cerebral tissue with "truly" normal MTR values accompanies the accumulation of irreversible disability, independently of the concomitant accumulation of MRI-visible lesions. In PPMS, this agrees with the frequent finding of diffuse T2 signal abnormalities in the brain and cervical cord [6]. In addition, in our sample of PPMS patients, average brain MTR values were only in part correlated with T2- and T1-visible lesion load. The correlation coefficients were about -0.3, indicating that less than 10% of MTR variability was explained by the burden of macroscopic lesions.

All of this suggests that NABT pathology in PPMS does not merely reflect wallerian degeneration of axons traversing macroscopic lesions [47], but might be related to the occurrence of multiple discrete lesions beyond the resolution of conventional scanning. This is consistent with the demonstration that in PPMS (1) individual T2-hyperintense lesions tend on average to be smaller in size than those seen in SPMS [3], and (2) diffuse blood-brain barrier leakage can occur independently of focal enhancing lesions [48]. Why, in PPMS patients, diffuse brain tissue damage develops with an evident disproportion between MRI-visible lesion burden and NABT pathology still remains an unresolved issue. Disappointingly, we did not find any correlation between individual brain or NABT MTR histogram-derived measures and patients' EDSS score. This could be mainly due to the limitations of the EDSS, including the fact that this scale is heavily weighted towards locomotor disability [38]. This is confirmed by the improved correlations obtained when cognitive scales [49] or composite scores [50] are used to assess neurological disability in PPMS.

Another potential useful application of MT MRI in the study of PPMS is to provide paraclinical markers of the disease evolution over time, with the ultimate aim of monitoring the efficacy of new experimental treatments. In a preliminary study, Filippi et al. [51] compared changes in T2 and T1 lesion load and brain and NABT MTR histogram-derived quantities over a period of 1 year in 96 patients with various MS phenotypes, including a subgroup of 9 with PPMS. Disappointingly, no significant changes in histographic quantities were observed in PPMS, while such changes were noted in SPMS patients. These data, although limited by the small size of the patient sample, seem to suggest that brain MT MRI-derived measures are not sensitive enough to conduct clinical trials with relatively short follow-up periods in patients with PPMS.

Cervical Cord

The technical difficulties in the acquisition of MT MRI scans from the cervical cord have recently been overcome and it is now feasible to obtain good-quality MTR maps from slabs of either sagittal or axial slices covering this region [36].

Cervical cord MTR histogram-derived metrics well differentiate MS patients from normal controls [36, 52, 53]. However, when RRMS patients are considered in isolation, cord MTR histogram characteristics are similar to those from healthy subjects [52]. That cervical cord MTR abnormalities might well reflect the presence of irreversible MS damage is confirmed by the results of two preliminary studies comparing cervical cord MTR histograms from RR, SP, and PP MS patients [52, 53]. Filippi et al. [52] found that PP and SP MS patients have similar cord histogram characteristics, even though less damage was apparent on the corresponding MRI scans of patients with PPMS. Lycklama à Nijeholt et al. [53] reported that combining cervical cord MTR and cross-sectional area values leads to a significant relationship with patients' EDSS scores ($r = -0.46$). In addition, the correlation between brain MRI lesion burden and average cervical cord MTR, as well as the correlations between brain and cord MTR histogram-derived quantities, have been found to be, at best, of moderate strength [54]. This indicates that the assessment of cervical cord damage using MTR histogram analysis can provide complementary information to that derived from the study of the brain, with the potential to increase our ability to explain the clinical manifestations of the disease.

The latter hypothesis has been investigated in our large-scale study comparing PP and SP MS [45], in which both brain and cervical cord MRI and MT MRI scans were obtained from all the patients and healthy controls. For the cervical cord, the number and burden of lesions and the cross-sectional area were assessed and MTR histogram analysis was performed. We found a similar burden of cervical cord lesions in PP and SP MS patients, contrary to what was seen for the brain [6, 7, 45]. This finding underpins the importance of MS pathology in the cord in patients with progressive accumulation of disability, independent of the way this occurs, i.e., with or without preceding or superimposed relapses. The modest inverse relationship we found between cord area and disease duration ($r = -0.25$) suggests that the development of cord atrophy might also be dependent upon the time elapsed from the clinical onset of MS. This is also confirmed by the more pronounced degree of cord area reduction found in SPMS patients, who had a longer average disease duration than PPMS patients, but similar levels of disability. Cord MTR histogram findings from both PP and SP MS patients were abnormal, but cord MTR histogram peak height was significantly lower in the latter group, suggesting a major reduction in the proportion of pixels belonging to truly normal tissue. The lack of significant correlations we found between MRI or MT MRI measures of MS pathology in the brain and cord suggests that degenerative processes affecting fiber tracts descending from brain lesions play only a modest role in determining the severity of PPMS-related cervical cord pathology. As in a previous study [53], we did not find a significant correlation between cord cross-sectional area and MTR histogram-derived quantities from the same region. This indicates that cord MTR histogram analysis encompasses both the loss of fibers leading to MRI-visible cord atrophy and the microscopic tissue damage affecting the remaining cord parenchyma [36, 52-54]. Similarly to what was found for the brain [45], we did not find any correlation between individual cord MRI or MT

MRI measures and patients' EDSS scores. Only by combining cord measures reflecting the severity of atrophy (cross-sectional area at C2 level) and that of intrinsic pathology in the remaining tissue (MTR histogram peak height) did we obtain a composite model with a relatively low ($r = 0.21$), but significant correlation with PPMS patients' EDSS score. This suggests that multiparametric MRI studies of the cervical cord, including MT MRI, might provide additional paraclinical measures of outcome for monitoring the evolution of PPMS.

DT MRI Studies

In the last few years, an increasing number of DT MRI studies has been conducted in MS [24-31, 33, 55]. However, only a few of these studies included PPMS patients [25, 26, 29, 33]. Droogan et al. [29] compared the DT MRI characteristics of 35 MS patients with various clinical phenotypes (9 patients were affected by PPMS). In this study, brain coverage was limited to four to six central slices and a ROI-based analysis of MS lesions and NAWM was performed. No significant differences were found between MS clinical subgroups as regards lesion or NAWM ADC and anisotropy indices, nor there was a correlation between DT MRI findings and patients' disability. These findings have been confirmed by another, more recent report [26], where a larger brain coverage (ten slices) was achieved and 30 PPMS patients were studied. In this study [26], PPMS patients showed significantly higher $\bar{D}$ and lower FA values than healthy controls in the NAWM at the levels of the corpus callosum and of the internal capsule, whereas this was not the case for RR and SP MS patients. In addition, no significant correlations were found between PPMS patients' EDSS scores and lesion or NAWM DT MRI findings, whereas in the SPMS group the strength of these correlations was moderate. These findings might indicate that, in PPMS, the loss of structural barriers to water motion in the internal capsule and the loss of fiber organization in the corpus callosum might contribute to the presence of severe locomotor disability and cognitive impairment, despite the paucity of MRI-visible abnormalities in these sites. In the study of Ciccarelli et al. [25], a DT MRI acquisition scheme allowing 21 brain slices to be obtained was used and ROI analysis of scans from 8 PPMS patients was performed in the NAGM of basal ganglia and cerebellum and in the infratentorial and supratentorial NAWM. Again, no significant differences were found between MS subgroups. In PPMS, only a significant correlation between EDSS score and infratentorial NAWM $\bar{D}$ was found. Cercignani et al. [33] created histograms of $\bar{D}$ and FA values from a large portion of the central brain (i.e., including both T2-visible lesions and NABT) from 30 PPMS patients. All the histogram-derived quantities showed significant differences between PPMS patients and healthy controls, but no differences were found among PP, RR, and SP MS patients. In addition, no significant correlations were found between DT MRI findings and PPMS patients' disability, contrary to what was seen for the other MS subgroups.

We have recently concluded [56] a large-scale DT MRI study where findings from 96 patients with PPMS were compared with those from SPMS patients and healthy subjects. In this study, we produced histograms of $\bar{D}$ and FA values from the brain tissue and, using a segmentation process based on FA thresholding [34], histograms of $\bar{D}$ values from the NAWM and NAGM in isolation. We found that the average lesion $\bar{D}$ was significantly higher in SP than in PP MS patients. Given this and the greater amount of brain tissue involved by T2-visible lesions in SPMS, in these patients the severity of intrinsic lesion damage might play an important role in the accumulation of irreversible disability. This agrees with longitudinal MT MRI data showing a progressive increase of tissue damage within newly formed lesions in patients with SPMS [57]. By contrast, the low amount of T2-visible lesions and the observation that the severity of intrinsic tissue damage within individual lesions is lower in PP than in SP MS suggest that other factors in addition to the presence of lesions affected by marked tissue disruption act in determining the dynamics of PPMS evolution. $\bar{D}$ and FA histogram analysis from brain tissue showed that, in PPMS patients, the histographic quantities were all significantly different from those of healthy subjects. The severity of brain tissue damage was, however, found to be greater in SP than in PP MS patients. Similarly to what was seen for brain MTR histograms [45], the results of group comparisons for $\bar{D}$ and FA histogram-derived quantities did not change after correction for subjects' brain volume, confirming that in MS patients the observed changes are not attributable to the inclusion of pixels with significant partial volume effects from the CSF. We found that both NAWM and NAGM $\bar{D}$ histogram-derived quantities were different between PPMS patients and age-matched healthy subjects. Again, tissue damage in both these brain compartments was more pronounced in SP than in PP MS patients. Although these results indicate a net loss and disorganization of structural barriers to water molecular motion in the NAWM, we can only speculate on the possible pathological substrates, and correlative studies are needed to clarify this issue. Nevertheless, subtle pathological changes are known to occur in the NAWM of patients with MS, including abnormally thin myelin and axonal loss [11], with the potential to cause increased $\bar{D}$ values. Our results also confirm that, in PPMS, brain NAGM is not spared by the pathological process. There are at least two factors which may contribute to the increased $\bar{D}$ values found in the NAGM of PPMS patients: first, the presence of discrete MS lesions, which go undetected when using T2-weighted imaging [58, 59], and, second, the presence of wallerian degeneration of gray matter neurons, secondary to the damage of fibers traversing MS white matter lesions [47]. However, the modest correlation ($r = 0.4$) we observed between macroscopic lesion load and average NAGM $\bar{D}$ suggests that the second mechanism is likely to account only for a limited part of DT MRI findings from the NAGM.

Conclusions

Several cross-sectional studies using either MT or DT MRI have consistently demonstrated that brain NAWM and NAGM are damaged in patients with PPMS. The functional relevance of this diffuse brain pathology is, however, still unclear.

MT MRI studies of the cervical cord indicate that, whereas brain MS pathology may have different patterns in PP and SP MS, cord damage plays an important role in determining the irreversible accumulation of MS disability, independent of the way this occurs. Large-scale longitudinal studies are now warranted to assess whether brain and cervical cord MT or DT MRI histogram analysis may be sensitive enough to detect the progression of PPMS pathology over time and to provide paraclinical measures of outcome for monitoring its evolution.

References

1. Thompson AJ, Polman CH, Miller DH et al (1997) Primary progressive multiple sclerosis. Brain 120:1085-1096
2. Cottrell DA, Kremenchutzky M, Rice GP et al (1999) The natural history of multiple sclerosis: a geographically based study. 5. The clinical features and natural history of primary progressive multiple sclerosis. Brain 122:625-639
3. Thompson AJ, Kermode AG, MacManus DG et al (1990) Patterns of disease activity in multiple sclerosis: clinical and magnetic resonance imaging study. Br Med J 300:631-634
4. Thompson AJ, Kermode AG, Wicks D et al (1991) Major differences in the dynamics of primary and secondary progressive multiple sclerosis. Ann Neurol 29:53-62
5. Kidd D, Thorpe JW, Kendall BE et al (1996) MRI dynamics of brain and spinal cord in progressive multiple sclerosis. J Neurol Neurosurg Psychiatry 60:15-19
6. Lycklama à Nijeholt GJ, van Walderveen MAA, Castelijns JA et al (1998) Brain and spinal cord abnormalities in multiple sclerosis. Correlation between MRI parameters, clinical subtypes and symptoms. Brain 121:687-697
7. Stevenson VL, Miller DH, Rovaris M et al (1999) Primary and transitional progressive MS. A clinical and MRI cross-sectional study. Neurology 52:839-845
8. van Walderveen MAA, Lycklama à Nijeholt GJ, Ader HJ et al (2001) Hypointense lesions on T1-weighted spin-echo magnetic resonance imaging. Relation to clinical characteristics in subgroups of patients with multiple sclerosis. Arch Neurol 58:76-81
9. Revesz T, Kidd D, Thompson AJ et al (1994) A comparison of the pathology of primary and secondary progressive multiple sclerosis. Brain 117:759-765
10. van Walderveen MAA, Kamphorst W, Scheltens P et al (1998) Histopathologic correlate of hypointense lesions on T_1-weighted spin-echo MRI in multiple sclerosis. Neurology 50:1282-1288
11. Allen IV, McKeown SR (1979) A histological, histochemical and biochemical study of the macroscopically normal white matter in multiple sclerosis. J Neurol Sci 41:81-89
12. Filippi M, Grossman RI, Comi G (eds) (1999) Magnetization transfer in multiple sclerosis. Neurology 53: Suppl 3
13. Cercignani M, Horsfield MA (2001) The physical basis of diffusion-weighted MRI. J Neurol Sci 186(Suppl 1):S11-S14
14. McDonald WI, Miller DH, Barnes D (1992) The pathological evolution of multiple sclerosis. Neuropathol Appl Neurobiol 18:319-334
15. Dousset V, Grossman RI, Ramer KN et al (1992) Experimental allergic encephalomyelitis and multiple sclerosis: lesion characterization with magnetization transfer imaging. Radiology 182:483-491
16. Dousset V, Brochet B, Vital A et al (1995) Lysolecithin-induced demyelination in pri-

mates: preliminary in vivo study with MR and magnetization transfer. AJNR Am J Neuroradiol 16:225-231

17. Deloire-Grassin MSA, Brochet B, Quesson B et al (2000) In vivo evaluation of remyelination in rat brain by magnetization transfer imaging. J Neurol Sci 178:10-16

18. van Waesberghe JH, Kamphorst W, DeGroot CJ et al (1999) Axonal loss in multiple sclerosis lesions: magnetic resonance imaging insights into substrates of disability. Ann Neurol 46:747-754

19. LeBihan D, Breton E, Lallemand D et al (1986) MR imaging of intravoxel incoherent motions: application to diffusion and perfusion in neurologic disorders. Radiology 161:401-407

20. Woessner DE (1963) NMR spin-echo self-diffusion measurement on fluids undergoing restricted diffusion. J Phys Chem 67:1365-1367

21. Le Bihan D, Turner R, Pekar J, Moonen CTW (1991) Diffusion and perfusion imaging by gradient sensitization: design, strategy and significance. J Magn Reson Imaging 1:7-8

22. Basser PJ, Mattiello J, LeBihan D (1994) MR diffusion tensor spectroscopy and imaging. Biophys J 66:259-267

23. Pierpaoli C, Basser PJ (1996) Towards a quantitative assessment of diffusion anisotropy. Magn Reson Med 36:893-906

24. Cercignani M, Iannucci G, Rocca MA et al (2000) Pathologic damage in MS assessed by diffusion-weighted and magnetization transfer MRI. Neurology 54:1139-1144

25. Ciccarelli O, Werring DJ, Wheeler-Kingshott CAM et al (2001) Investigation of MS normal-appearing brain using diffusion tensor MRI with clinical correlations. Neurology 56:926-933

26. Filippi M, Cercignani M, Inglese M et al (2001) Diffusion tensor magnetic resonance imaging in multiple sclerosis. Neurology 56:304-311

27. Filippi M, Iannucci G, Cercignani M et al (2000) A quantitative study of water diffusion in MS lesions and NAWM using echo-planar imaging. Arch Neurol 57:1017-1021

28. Werring DJ, Clark CA, Barker GJ et al (1999) Diffusion tensor imaging of lesions and normal-appearing white matter in multiple sclerosis. Neurology 52:1626-1632

29. Droogan AG, Clark CA, Werring DJ et al (1999) Comparison of multiple sclerosis clinical subgroups using navigated spin echo diffusion-weighted imaging. Magn Reson Imaging 17:653-661

30. Rocca MA, Cercignani M, Iannucci G et al (2000) Weekly diffusion-weighted imaging study of NAWM in MS. Neurology 55:882-884

31. Bammer R, Augustin M, Strasser-Fuchs S et al (2000) Magnetic resonance diffusion tensor imaging for characterizing diffuse and focal white matter abnormalities in multiple sclerosis. Magn Reson Med 44:583-591

32. van Buchem MA, McGowan JC, Kolson DL et al (1996) Quantitative volumetric magnetization transfer analysis in multiple sclerosis: estimation of macroscopic and microscopic disease burden. Magn Reson Med 36:632-636

33. Cercignani M, Inglese M, Pagani E et al (2001) Mean diffusivity and fractional anisotropy histograms of patients with multiple sclerosis. AJNR Am J Neuroradiol 22:952-958

34. Cercignani M, Bozzali M, Iannucci G et al (2001) Magnetisation transfer ratio and mean diffusivity of normal appearing white and grey matter from patients with multiple sclerosis. J Neurol Neurosurg Psychiatry 70:311-317

35. Miller DH, Leary S, Dehmeshki J et al (2001) Evidence for grey matter involvement in primary progressive MS: a magnetization transfer imaging study (abstract). J Neurol 248 (Suppl 2):27

36. Bozzali M, Rocca MA, Iannucci G, Pereira C, Comi G, Filippi M (1999) Magnetization transfer histogram analysis of the cervical cord in patients with multiple sclerosis. AJNR Am J Neuroradiol 20:1803-1808
37. Gass A, Barker GJ, Kidd D et al (1994) Correlation of magnetization transfer ratio with clinical disability in multiple sclerosis. Ann Neurol 36:62-67
38. Kurtzke JF (1983) Rating neurological impairment in multiple sclerosis: an expanded disability status scale (EDSS). Neurology 33:1444-1452
39. Leary SM, Davie CA, Parker GJM et al (1999) ^{1}H magnetic resonance spectroscopy of normal appearing white matter in primary progressive multiple sclerosis. J Neurol 246:1023-1026
40. Filippi M, Iannucci G, Tortorella C et al (1999) Comparison of MS clinical phenotypes using conventional and magnetization transfer MRI. Neurology 52:588-594
41. Dehmeshki J, Silver NC, Leary SM et al (2001) Magnetisation transfer ratio histogram analysis of primary progressive and other multiple sclerosis subgroups. J Neurol Sci 185:11-17
42. Lublin FD, Reingold SC, the National Multiple Sclerosis Society (USA) Advisory Committee on Clinical Trials of New Agents in Multiple Sclerosis (1996) Defining the clinical course of multiple sclerosis: results of an international survey. Neurology 46:907-911
43. Tortorella C, Viti B, Bozzali M et al (2000) A magnetization transfer histogram study of normal-appearing brain tissue in MS. Neurology 54:186-193
44. Bozzali M, Cercignani M, Comi G, Filippi M (2001) Gray matter involvement in different multiple sclerosis phenotypes: a diffusion tensor and magnetization transfer imaging study (abstract). Proc Int Soc Magn Reson Med 9:95
45. Rovaris M, Bozzali M, Santuccio G et al (2001) *In vivo* assessment of the brain and cervical cord pathology of patients with primary progressive multiple sclerosis. Brain 124:2540-2549
46. Thompson AJ, Montalban X, Barkhof F (2000) Diagnostic criteria for primary progressive multiple sclerosis: a position paper. Ann Neurol 47:831-835
47. Evangelou N, Konz D, Esiri MM et al (2000) Regional axonal loss in the corpus callosum correlates with cerebral white matter lesion volume and distribution in multiple sclerosis. Brain 123:1845-1849
48. Silver NC, Tofts PS, Symms MR et al (2001) Quantitative contrast-enhanced magnetic resonance imaging to evaluate blood-brain barrier integrity in multiple sclerosis: a preliminary study. Mult Scler 7:75-82
49. Camp SJ, Stevenson VL, Thompson AJ et al (1999) Cognitive function in primary progressive and transitional progressive multiple sclerosis. A controlled study with MRI correlates. Brain 122:1341-1348
50. Tintorè M, Brieva L, Rovira A et al (2001) Primary progressive multiple sclerosis: a clinical and MRI cross-sectional study using T2-lesion load, total brain parenchymal fraction and spinal cord cross-sectional area (abstract). J Neurol 248 (Suppl 2):136
51. Filippi M, Inglese M, Rovaris M et al (2000) Magnetization transfer imaging to monitor the evolution of MS: a one-year follow up study. Neurology 55:940-946
52. Filippi M, Bozzali M, Horsfield MA et al (2000) A conventional and magnetization transfer MRI study of the cervical cord in patients with MS. Neurology 54:207-213
53. Lycklama à Nijeholt GJ, Castelijns JA, Lazeron RH et al (2000) Magnetization transfer ratio of the spinal cord in multiple sclerosis: relationship to atrophy and neurologic disability. J Neuroimaging 10:67-72

54. Rovaris M, Bozzali M, Santuccio G et al (2000) Relative contributions of brain and cervical cord pathology to multiple sclerosis disability: a study with magnetisation transfer ratio analysis. J Neurol Neurosurg Psychiatry 69:723-727

55. Wilson M, Morgan PS, Lin X et al (2001) Quantitative diffusion weighted magnetic resonance imaging, cerebral atrophy and disability in multiple sclerosis. J Neurol Neurosurg Psychiatry 70:318-322

56. Santuccio G, Bozzali M, Rovaris M et al (2001) In vivo study of CNS tissue damage in patients with primary progressive MS (abstract). Neurology 56 [Suppl 3]:A379

57. Rocca MA, Mastronardo G, Rodegher M et al (1999) Long-term changes of magnetization transfer-derived measures from patients with relapsing-remitting and secondary progressive multiple sclerosis. AJNR Am J Neuroradiol 20:821-827

58. Kidd D, Barkhof F, McConnell R et al (1999) Cortical lesions in multiple sclerosis. Brain 122:17-26

59. Brownell B, Hughes JT (1962) The distribution of plaques in the cerebrum in multiple sclerosis. J Neurol Neurosurg Psychiatry 25:315-320

Chapter 9

Proton Magnetic Resonance Spectroscopy

Z. Caramanos, A.C. Santos, S.J. Francis, S. Narayanan, D. Pelletier, D.L. Arnold

Introduction

Primary Progressive Multiple Sclerosis

Approximately 85%-90% of patients with multiple sclerosis (MS) will begin their disease with a course of relapses and remissions and are therefore classified as having relapsing-remitting (RR) MS [1]. Some of these patients will eventually go on to develop a progressive disability that is characterized by a slow, irreversible deterioration over time, at which point they will be classified as having secondary progressive (SP) MS [1]. Interestingly, about 10%-15% of patients experience a progressive course, without any relapses or remissions, from the onset of their disease, and they are classified as having primary progressive (PP) MS [2].

The pathological hallmark of all subtypes of MS is the presence of demyelinating lesions that are focal, inflammatory, and appear hyperintense on T2-weighted magnetic resonance imaging (MRI) [3]. Importantly, however, it has been shown that the nonlesional, normal-appearing white matter (NAWM) of MS patients (i.e., white matter that appears normal on gross pathological inspection) can also demonstrate various microscopic abnormalities [4-6].

Despite the relative severity of their functional disability – usually assessed with the Kurtzke Expanded Disability Status Scale (EDSS) [7] – patients with PPMS typically present with less-severe findings on conventional MRI of the brain. On average, relative to equally-disabled patients with SPMS, patients with PPMS: (1) present with fewer lesions and a smaller total lesion load [8, 9], (2) develop fewer lesions over time despite a clear increase in disability [10], and (3) show less gadolinium enhancement in those lesions that they do have [11]. PPMS patients also typically present with (4) a lesser degree of brain atrophy as well as (5) abnormalities that are more diffuse [12]. A similar pattern of results has also been found in the spinal cords of PPMS versus SPMS patients. For example, despite having similar EDSS values, PPMS patients have, on average, (6) significantly fewer spinal cord lesions and (7) significantly less spinal cord atrophy [9]. As recently suggested by Leary et al. [13], the marked disparity between the clinical deterioration seen in PPMS patients and their findings on conventional MRI may well reflect a different mechanism of irrecoverable neurological deficit in this group: for example, the neurological deficits associated with the RR stage of the disease might reflect the effects of demyelination, whereas those associated with progressive-disease deficits might reflect progressive axonal loss (which in PPMS – as opposed to SPMS – might be present from early in the course of the disease [14]).

Proton Magnetic Resonance Spectroscopy

Although conventional MRI shows great sensitivity in detecting MS lesions, it is unable to detect dysfunction of neurons and their axonal processes directly. On the other hand, as recently reviewed by Arnold et al. [15], the various approaches to in vivo proton magnetic resonance spectroscopy (^{1}H-MRS) can provide specific information regarding neuronal and axonal integrity. These approaches include: (1) single-voxel ^{1}H-MRS studies (in which proton spectra are acquired from a single volume) and (2) ^{1}H-MRS imaging studies [^{1}H-MRSI, in which proton spectra are obtained from multiple volume elements (i.e., voxels) at the same time].

Metabolites Measured

Although fundamentally similar to conventional MRI (which is based on the mapping of protons associated with water), ^{1}H-MRS is different in that it records signals from other metabolites that are present in brain tissue but that, generally, can only be measured when the signal from water is suppressed. Importantly, this metabolic information can provide chemical and pathological specificity that is not available from conventional MRI [16]. As shown in Fig. 1, the water-suppressed, localized ^{1}H-MRS spectrum of the normal human brain reveals three major resonance peaks, the locations of which are expressed as the difference in parts per million (ppm) between the resonance frequency of the compound of interest and that of a standard (tetramethylsilane). These peaks are commonly ascribed to the following metabolites: (1) tetramethyl amines (Cho), which resonate at 3.2 ppm and are mostly choline-containing phospholipids that participate in membrane synthesis and degradation; (2) creatine and phosphocreatine (Cr), which resonate at 3.0 ppm and play an important role in energy metabolism; and (3) N-acetyl groups (NA), which resonate at 2.0 ppm and are comprised primarily of the neuronally-localized compound N-acetylaspartate (NAA).

Methods of Quantification

Whereas precise absolute quantification of these resonance intensities is more complicated in vivo than it is with in vitro ^{1}H-MRS, various methods have been developed to provide semiabsolute quantification of ^{1}H-MRS and ^{1}H-MRSI data acquired in vivo. These include (1) the use of an *external reference* (e.g., a phantom) with known metabolite concentrations – the most widely-used approach being the LCModel method, which considers the [1]H-MR spectra arising from tissues acquired in vivo as a linear combination of spectra arising from known metabolite solutions acquired in vitro [19]; and (2) the use of an *internal reference* to correct for various external inhomogeneities that affect metabolite resonance intensities – the most widely used reference being the water signal arising

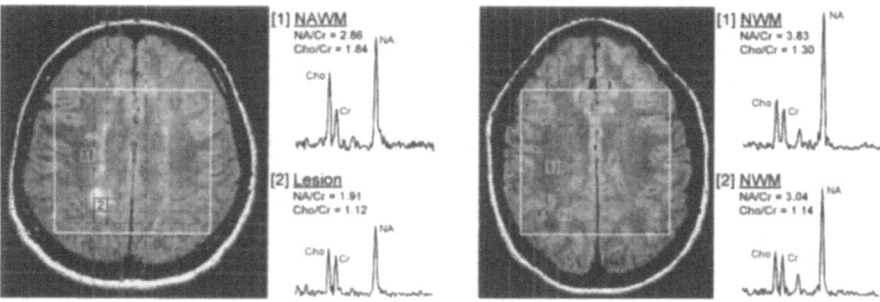

Fig. 1. Proton-density-weighted magnetic resonance images through the centrum semiovale, as well as the results of ¹H-MRSI, in one of our patients with primary progressive multiple sclerosis (*left*) and in one of our normal control subjects (*right*). Methods: For each individual, combined proton MRI and MRSI examinations of the brain were obtained in a single session for each examination using a scanner operating at 1.5 T (Philips Gyroscan; Philips Medical Systems, Best, the Netherlands). Two-dimensional ¹H-MRSI scans were obtained using a 90°-180°-180° pulse sequence (TR 2000 ms, TE 272 ms, 32 × 32 phase-encoding steps with 1 signal average per step, and a 250-mm field of view), the effective spatial resolution being about 12 × 12 × 20 mm after k-space filtering. These methods are presented in more detail elsewhere [17, 18]. ¹H-MRSI findings: The *superimposed grid* in each image represents the ¹H-MRSI voxels, and the *large, thick, white box* represents the ¹H-MRSI volume of interest for that individual. The *smaller, numbered boxes* represent voxels of normal-appearing white matter (NAWM) and lesional brain tissue in the patient and normal white matter (NWM) in the normal control subject. The ¹H-MRSI spectra from within each of these voxels is shown to the *right* of each image. The areas under the NA and Cho peaks (normalized to Cr) are shown above each spectrum. The spectra have been scaled so that the Cr peak in each of them is the same height

from cerebrospinal fluid (CSF) [20, 21]. Note that, whereas the internal reference approach can be used in both single-voxel ¹H-MRS and ¹H-MRSI studies, the external reference approach is difficult to adapt to ¹H-MRSI and has only been used in single-voxel ¹H-MRS.

Another method, which is much simpler and can also be used in ¹H-MRSI studies, is to normalize the NA and Cho signal intensities to the signal intensity from Cr in the same voxel [15]. Of course, this latter method does not provide absolute quantification and, importantly, the resulting measures of relative concentration are only valid if the underlying pathology does not substantially affect the local concentration of Cr. Some investigators have suggested that Cr is a putative marker of gliosis [22, 23]; however, as reviewed elsewhere [15], Cr concentrations have been shown to be relatively constant in both the lesions [24, 25] and the NAWM [25, 26] of patients with MS.

Metabolites of Interest in MS

In the mature mammalian brain, NAA appears to be located exclusively in neurons and neuronal processes [27]. The resonance from NA has proved to be extremely useful for the characterization of pathology in MS, and the ratio of NA to Cr has been used to quantify neuronal and axonal integrity in vivo in patients with MS for over a decade now [17, 28]. Importantly, the validity of NA as a surrogate for axonal density in MS has recently been confirmed directly in a study that combined in vivo ^{1}H-MRS and histopathologic analysis of subsequent biopsy specimens from the same individuals [29]. As recently reviewed by Arnold et al. [15], the Cho resonance peak can also provide useful information related to myelin breakdown, and in MS it has been shown to rise early in the course of plaque evolution and to sometimes stay elevated for months or years afterwards [25, 30].

Aims of the Present Chapter

If it is true that the functional disabilities observed in PPMS reflect a progressive axonal loss that is present from early in the course of that form of MS, it might be informative to examine the ^{1}H-MRS findings in patients with PPMS and compare and contrast them with those in normal controls as well as with those in patients with the RR and SP forms of the disease. The rest of this chapter is, thus, devoted to reviewing the findings in the literature that have used some form of ^{1}H-MRS to study patients with PPMS.

Literature Review

Studies Reviewed

As of the time of writing (July 2001), we found 12 different studies that used some form of ^{1}H-MRS or ^{1}H-MRSI to study patients with PPMS [13, 31-41]. Of these 12 studies, only 7 were articles published in peer-reviewed journals [13, 31, 32, 34, 35, 37, 41], the other 5 being abstracts published as part of the conference proceedings of the International Society for Magnetic Resonance in Medicine [33, 36, 38, 39] or the American Academy of Neurology [40]. Information regarding the general methodology used in each of these studies is presented in Table 1.

In Vitro ^{1}H-MRS Studies of CSF in Patients with MS

The first ^{1}H-MRS study that included PPMS patients was an ex vivo investigation that used in vitro high-resolution ^{1}H-MRS to examine the CSF in patients with either RRMS ($n = 13$) or PPMS ($n = 6$) as compared to diseased controls [31]. These controls ($n = 17$) had undergone a lumbar puncture but did not turn out to suffer from any inflammatory, degenerative, or tumoral disease of the central nervous system. The MS patients were studied prior to any treatment with corticosteroids and their CSF was found to have a very moderate metabolic alteration relative to the control patients as reflected in: (1) increased mean concentrations of lactate and fructose in both MS groups, (2) decreased mean concentrations of creatinine and phenylalanine in both MS groups, and (3) decreased mean concen-

Table 1. Methods used in proton magnetic resonance spectroscopy (¹H-MRS) studies of patients with primary progressive multiple sclerosis

Study	Scanner model (magnet strength)	TR / TE	¹H-MRS study (voxel size)	Measure quantified (units)	Metabolites measured	Tissues studied	Groups studied
Nicoli et al. 1996 [31]	Bruker AM 400-WB (9.4 T)	3160 / n.d.	In vitro 1-D High-resolution scan	Absolute concentration (mM)	31 metabolites[a]	CSF	DC, PP, RR
Davie et al. 1997 [32]	GE Signa (1.5 T)	2000 / 135	Single voxel (3.5 - 6.0 ml)	CSF-water-normalized concentration (mM)	NA, Cr, Cho	Lesions and NAWM	NC, PP, RR, SP, BD
Pan et al. 1998[b] [33]	n.d. (4.5 T)	2000 / 50	2-D imaging (1.1 ml)	CSF-water-normalized concentration (mM)	NA, Cr, Cho	PVWM and Cortical gray matter	NC, PP, RR
Pike et al. 1999 [34]	Philips Gyroscan ACS II (1.5 T)	2000 / 272	2-D imaging (1.2 ml)	Cr-normalized peak areas (ratios)	NA/Cr	Lesions	PP, RR, SP
Leary et al. 1999 [13]	GE Signa Horizon Echospeed (1.5 T)	3000 / 30	Single voxel (1.0- 3.2 ml)	LCModel-calculated [19] concentrations (mM)	NA, NAA, Cr NA/Cr, NAA/Cr	NAWM	NC, PP
Cucurella et al. 2000 [35]	Siemens Magnetom-Vision (1.5 T)	1600 / 135	Single voxel (2 × 2 × 2 cm)	VARPRO [44] time-domain-fitted values (AU)	NA, Cho, Cr NA/Cr, Cho/Cr	Lesions and NAWM	NC, PP, SP[c]
Suhy et al. 2000 [37]	Siemens Magnetom-Vision (1.5 T)	1800 / 135	Single voxel (2.4 ml)	CSF-water-normalized values (AU)	NA, Cr, Cho NA/Cr	Lesions and NAWM	NC, PP, RR
Pan et al. 2000[b] [36]	Varian Siemens Inova (1.5 T)	2000 / 50	2-D imaging (0.64 ml)	CSF-water-wormalized values (mM)	NA, Cr, Cho	PVWM	PP, RR, SP[d]
Oh et al. 2001[b] [38]	GE Medical system Signa (1.5 T)	1000 / 144	2-D Imaging (1.5 ml)	Cr-normalized peak areas (ratios)	NA/Cr, Cho/Cr	Corpus callosum	NC, PP, RR, SP[d]
Pelletier et al. 2001[b][39]	GE (1.5 T)	2000 / 144	3-D EPSI (0.56 ml)	Cr-normalized peak areas (ratios)	NA/Cr	Non-tissue-specific brain volumes	NC, PP, RR, SP
Pelletier et al. 2001[b] [40]	GE (1.5 T)	2000 / 144	3-D EPSI (0.56 ml)	Cr-normalized peak areas (ratios)	NA/Cr, Cho/Cr	Non-tissue-specific brain volumes	NC, PP[e]
Viala et al. 2001 [41]	GE Signa 5X (1.5 T)	1500 / 136	Single voxel (5.0-7.0 ml)	Cr-normalized peak areas (ratios)	NA/Cr, Cho/Cr	Lesions	PP, RR, SP[d]

TR, time to repetition (in ms); *TE*, time to echo (in ms); *n.d.*, no data (not specified in original report); *CSF*, cerebrospinal fluid; *DC*, diseased controls; *NC*, normal controls; *PP*, primary progressive multiple sclerosis (*MS*); *RR*, relapsing-remitting MS; *SP*, secondary progressive MS; *BD*, benign disease; *NA*, N-acetyl groups; *NAA*, N-acetylaspartate; *Cr*, creatine plus phosphocreatine; *Cho*, choline-containing phospholipids and other tetramethyl amines; *NAWM*, normal-appearing white matter; *PVWM*, periventricular white matter; *EPSI*, echo planar spectroscopic imaging [43]; *AU*, arbitrary units
[a] These metabolites included lactate, creatine, as well as three different NAA compounds
[b] These studies were published only in the form of an abstract
[c] Lesion and NAWM data were collected in separate samples of patients for this study
[d] These studies did not present their PPMS patients' data separately from that of their other subgroups
[e] PP subjects included a high- and a low-lesion load subgroup

trations of citrate in the RRMS group. Importantly, however, no differences were found between the two MS groups in their mean concentrations of any of the 31 metabolite resonances that were examined (which included three NAA metabolite resonances). Thus, the authors of this study concluded that RRMS and PPMS patients could not be distinguished on the basis of metabolic alterations detected by high-resolution ^{1}H-MRS of their CSF.

In Vivo ^{1}H-MRS Studies of Patients with MS

The remaining 11 studies [13, 32-41] all used an in vivo approach to study patients with PPMS as well as patients with other forms of MS, normal controls, or both. Unfortunately, two of the abstracts [36, 38] did not present ^{1}H-MRS data from the different MS subgroups separately and, thus, findings in patients with PPMS could not be compared to those in patients with other forms of the disease. Furthermore, one study [41], which did present data separately for RRMS and SPMS patients, did not present any data for the PPMS patients that had been examined (probably because there were only two patients with PPMS in that study). Whereas Pike et al. [34] did not present their ^{1}H-MRSI data broken down by MS subgroup, this information could be reconstructed from the figures that were provided. Thus, in total, eight studies presented some kind of ^{1}H-MRS or ^{1}H-MRSI data acquired from the brains of patients with PPMS. Information regarding the subjects included in these studies (as well those included in the study by Nicoli et al. [31] described above) is presented in Table 2. Findings from these studies that relate to subjects' NA, Cho, and Cr resonance intensities (quantified either semiabsolutely or relative to Cr) are described and summarized below.

NA-Related Findings

NA in Lesions
Three studies provided semiabsolute quantification of NA in the lesional brain-tissue of PPMS patients [32, 35, 37] (Fig. 2) and all three had consistent findings:
1. In 1997, Davie et al. [32] found that, in their groups of PPMS, RRMS, and SPMS patients, lesions that were large (i.e., 3.5-6.0 ml, large enough to minimize partial volume effects) and chronic (i.e., unchanged for at least 6 months) had lower median NA values than that measured in the white matter of their normal controls. As can be seen in Fig. 2, although differences amongst their three MS subgroups were not tested statistically, they did all have similar median lesional NA values. In this study, patients with "benign MS" (i.e., in this case, patients with RRMS of at least 10 years' duration and an EDSS score of 3.0 or less) were also studied and, interestingly, no difference was found between their median within-lesion NA value and that found within the controls' white matter. It should be noted, however, that the lesions in these patients with benign disease may have been smaller and, thus, this observation may have been more prone to partial volume effects.

Table 2. Table summarizing the subjects included in proton magnetic resonance spectroscopy (¹H-MRS) studies of patients with primary progressive multiple sclerosis

Study	Group	Subjects n	Subjects F/M	Descriptive statistics	Age (years)	EDSS	Disease duration
Nicoli et al. 1996 [31]	DC	17	1/16	Mean (SD)	47.4 (1.78)	n.d.	n.d.
	PP	6	6/0	"	52.2 (14.7)	n.d.	n.d.
	RR	13	12/1	"	29.5 (13.8)		
Davie et al. 1997 [32]	NC	9	n.d.	Median [range]	40 [18-57]		
	PP	8	n.d.	"	42 [37-47]	6 [5-7.5]	4.5 [1.5-19]
	RR	9	n.d.	"	31 [26-49]	3.5 [2-5.5]	3 [1-12]
	SP	10	n.d.	"	46 [21-55]	7 [4-8]	13.5 [5-25]
	BD	9	n.d.	"	45 [39-63]	2.5 [1-3]	20 [10-35]
Pan et al. 1998 [33]	NC	7	n.d.	n.d.	n.d.		
	PP	4	n.d.	Mean	n.d.	6.0-6.5	n.d.
	RR	4	n.d.	"	n.d.	< 1.5	n.d.
Pike et al. 1999 [34]	PP	5	1/4	Mean (SD) [range]	45 (10)	6 (1) [4-7]	n.d.
	RR	11	5/6	"	33 (6)	5 (1) [3-7]	n.d.
	SP	14	5/9	"	50 (8)	6 (1) [4-8]	n.d.
Leary et al. 1999 [13]	NC	16	n.d.	Mean [range]	46 [31-62]		
	PP	24	n.d.	Medianª [range]	481 [33-59]	4.5 [2.0-7.0]	6 [2-19]
Cucurella et al. 2000ᵇ [35] NAWM patients	NC	17	8/9	Mean (SD) [range]	46 (12.8) [21-64]		
	PP	11	4/7	"	47.4 (9.9) [32-67]	5.1 (1.8) [2-8.5]	9.5 (3.6) [4-15]
	SP	7	4/3	"	43.6 (13.0) [26-60]	6.1 (0.7) [4.5-6.5]	12.5 (5.4) [5-19]
Lesion patients	PP	6	5/1	"	44.2 (9.0) [32-55]	6 (1.8) [3.5-8]	10.8 (7) [6-24]
	SP	11	10/1	"	45.4 (9.1) [31-59]	5.3 (1.1) [4-6.5]	19.6 (12.9) [5-47]

cont.

Table 2. *Cont.*

Study	Group	Subjects n	F / M	Descriptive statistics	Age (years)	EDSS	Disease duration
Suhy et al. 2000 [37]	NC	20	7 / 13	Mean [range]	41.3 [25-49]		
	PP	15	5 / 10	Mean	47.5	4.4	9.07
	RR	13	6 / 7	"	39.5	2.5	7.79
Pelletier et al. 2001 [39]	NC	10	n.d.	[Range]	[21-55]		
	PP	8	n.d.	n.d.	n.d.	n.d.	n.d.
	RR	9	n.d.	n.d.	n.d.	n.d.	n.d.
	SP	21	n.d.	n.d.	n.d.	n.d.	n.d.
Pelletier et al. 2001 [40]	NC	10	n.d.	Mean (SD)	42.7 (9.3)		
High lesion load	PP	8	n.d.c	c	n.d.c	n.d.c	n.d.c
Low lesion load	PP	9	n.d.c	c	n.d.c	n.d.c	n.d.c

DC, diseased controls; *NC*, normal controls; *PP*, primary progressive multiple sclerosis (MS); *RR*, relapsing-remitting MS; *SP*, secondary progressive MS; *BD*, benign disease; *n*, total sample size; *F*, females; *M*, males; *SD*, standard deviation; *n.d*, no data (not specified in original report); *NAWM*, normal-appearing white matter

[a]Mean value given for age

[b]Lesion and NAWM data were collected in separate samples of patients for this study

[c] Although they did not present any descriptive statistics, the authors stated that their high- and low-lesion load subgroups did not differ with regard to their gender ratios or to their mean ages, EDSS scores, or disease durations

NA in Lesions

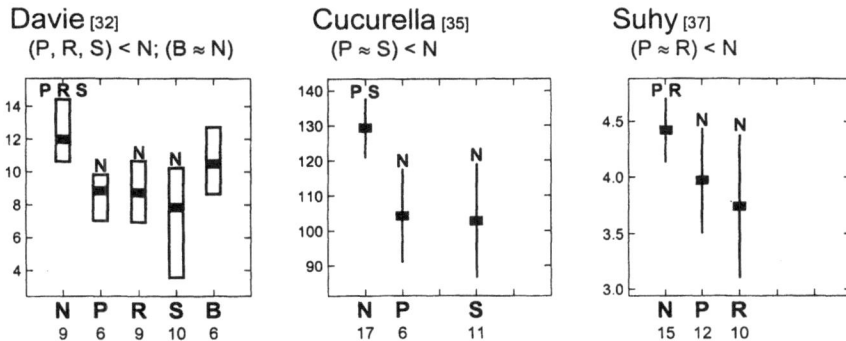

Fig. 2. Results of studies that quantified *N*-acetyl (NA) group resonance intensities in the lesional brain-tissue of patients with primary progressive (*P*), relapsing-remitting (R), secondary progressive (*S*), or benign (*B*) multiple sclerosis, as well as in the normal white matter tissue of normal control subjects (*N*); the numbers underneath each group signify sample size. For each study, the *heavy horizontal lines* and *surrounding boxes* signify group medians and ranges, whereas the *heavy horizontal lines* and *extending thin vertical lines* signify group means and standard deviations (depending on the descriptive statistics that were presented in the original publication). The *small letters* above each of the boxes and vertical lines signify which, if any, groups a particular group differed from in a statistically-significant sense (as presented in the original publication; all $p < 0.05$, although not necessarily corrected for the number of comparisons performed). ≈ in the statistical difference summaries above the plots signifies a lack of statistically-significant group differences. When groups are separated by a comma, the difference between the central-tendencies of those groups was not tested statistically. See Tables 1 and 2 for more information on the individual studies

2. In 2000, Cucurella et al. [35] found that the mean NA values measured within large (i.e., 8-ml cubes) and chronic (i.e., present for at least 4 months) lesions in the brains of their PPMS and SPMS patients did not differ from one another; furthermore, these values were both lower than those found in the normal white matter of their normal controls.
3. Similarly, in 2000, Suhy et al. [37] found that the lesion-containing voxels of their PPMS and RRMS patients had similar mean NA values, mean values that were lower than those seen in the spatially-analogous periventricular white matter of their normal controls.

NA in NAWM

Four studies provided semiabsolute quantification of NA in the NAWM of PPMS patients [13, 32, 35, 37] (Fig. 3). Again, all four had consistent findings. For example, although it was not possible for Davie et al. [32] to collect data from the NAWM of their RRMS and SPMS patients, they did find that, as for their lesion data, (1) the median NA-value in the NAWM of their benign-disease patients did

NA in NAWM

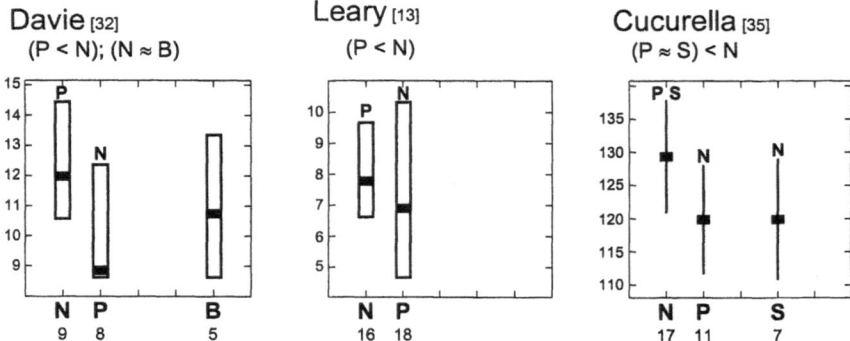

Fig. 3. Results of studies that quantified NA group resonance intensities in the NAWM of patients with primary progressive (*P*), relapsing-remitting (*R*), secondary progressive (*S*), or benign (*B*) multiple sclerosis, as well as in the normal white matter tissue of normal controls (*N*). See Fig. 2 legend for more information

not differ statistically from that of the white matter in their normal controls, and (2) there was a significant reduction in the NAWM NA values of their PPMS patients. Similarly, in 1999, Leary et al. [13] found that NA in the NAWM voxels of their PPMS patients was reduced relative to controls. Furthermore, Cucurella et al. [35] found equally-reduced NA values in the NAWM of their PPMS and SPMS patients. Finally, Suhy et al. [37] found equally-reduced values in their PPMS and RRMS patients. It should be noted that Cucurella et al. [35] tested and, as might be predicted, found that NA was less reduced in the NAWM than in the lesional brain tissue of both their PPMS and their SPMS patients (Figs. 2, 3).

In their study, Leary et al. [13] also tried to look specifically at NA. They found exactly the same results as they did for NA (i.e., reduced NAA values in the NAWM voxels of their PPMS patients, results not shown in Fig. 3).

NA in Periventricular White Matter and Gray Matter

In 1998, Pan and Whitaker [33] used ^{1}H-MRSI to provide semiabsolute quantification of NA in the periventricular white matter (PVWM) and the parietooccipital gray matter of PPMS and RRMS patients and normal controls (five ^{1}H-MRSI voxels of each tissue type per person). As shown in Fig. 4, their PPMS patients had a lower mean NA value in their PVWM voxels than did their RRMS patients. Although the difference between their patient groups and their normal control group was not tested statistically, it seems as though the RRMS patients had normal levels of PVWM NA and that the PPMS patients had reduced levels. This pattern seems to hold for the gray matter voxels as well (unfortunately no statistical results were presented in regard to the gray matter data). It should be noted, however, that the RRMS patients in the study by Pan and Whitaker had a very low level

NA in PVWM

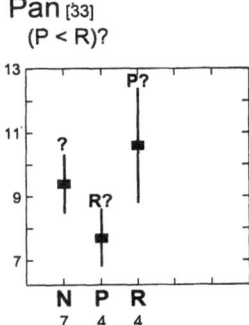

NA in Grey Matter

Fig. 4. Results of a study that quantified NA group resonance intensities in the periventricular white matter (PVWM) and occipitoparietal gray matter of patients with primary progressive (*P*) or relapsing-remitting (*R*) multiple sclerosis, as well as in the white matter and gray matter of normal controls (*N*). ? signifies the lack of an explicit statistical comparison in the original publication. See Fig. 2 legend for more information

of disability (i.e., EDSS < 1.5), which may explain why these patients' NA values seem to be relatively normal (e.g., similar to those of the benign MS group in the study by Davie et al. [32]. It should also be noted that this study included very few patients and, thus, these findings need to be replicated in a larger sample before they can be given much weight.

Cr-Related Findings

Cr in Lesions
Three studies provided semiabsolute quantification of Cr in the lesional brain-tissue of PPMS patients [32, 35, 37] (Fig. 5). For this resonance peak, the results were not as consistent as for the NA-related findings both Davie et al. [32] and Cucurella et al. [35] found that the average Cr values measured in their patients' lesion-containing voxels did not differ from those measured in their normal control subjects' white matter voxels. On the other hand, Suhy et al. [37] found that, whereas the mean Cr value was unchanged in their RRMS patients' lesions, the lesion voxels in their PPMS patients had a significantly-higher mean Cr value. One possible explanation for this finding is that Suhy et al. found a strong and significant, positive linear relationship between age and Cr values measured in their 20 normal controls ($Cr = 0.0136 \times age + 1.613, r = 0.77, p < 0.001$) but not in their patients – who had equally high values at all ages, regardless of group (RRMS: $Cr = -0.0006 \times age + 2.240$; PPMS: $Cr = -0.0031 \times age + 2.549$). In order to correct for this, they used linear-model age-corrected data for their normal controls, something that the other studies did not. It is important to note, however, that

Cr in Lesions

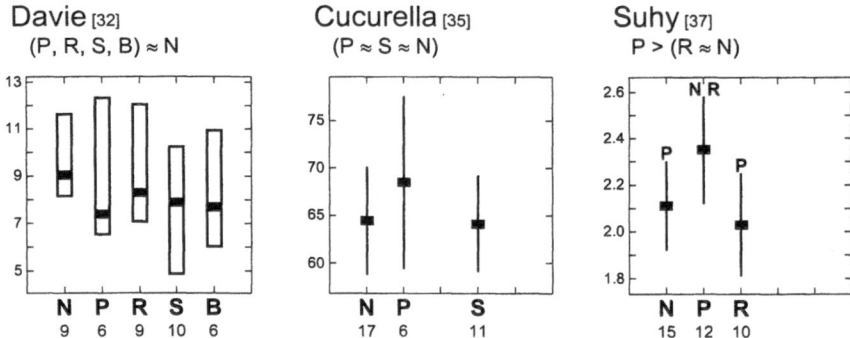

Fig. 5. Results of studies that quantified creatine plus phosphocreatine (Cr) resonance intensities in the lesional brain-tissue of patients with primary progressive (*P*), relapsing-remitting (*R*), secondary progressive (*S*), or benign (*B*) multiple sclerosis, as well as in the normal white matter tissue of normal controls (*N*). See Fig. 2 legend for more information. Note that the normal control data in the Suhy et al. study [37] are controlled for age (see text)

while the use of absolute quantification has certain advantages, it also requires various precise measurements and depends upon certain assumptions that combine to produce uncertain sources of variance. For example, in the study by Suhy et al. [37], individuals' metabolite values (including that of Cr) were normalized to their CSF signals on proton-density-weighted MRI. Importantly, this particular CSF signal is relatively low and, thus, susceptible to noise; therefore, this normalization may have been suboptimal.

Cr in NAWM

Four studies provided semiabsolute quantification of Cr in the NAWM of PPMS patients [13, 32, 35, 37] (Fig. 6). As was the case for the lesional tissue, this set of Cr findings was similarly inconsistent: Davie et al. [32], Leary et al. [13], and Cucurella et al. [35] all found that the average Cr values measured in their patients' NAWM voxels did not differ from those measured in their control subjects' white matter voxels. Once again, however, Suhy et al. [37] found that the mean Cr value in their PPMS patients' NAWM voxels was higher than that in their RRMS patients and was also higher than the age-corrected values in their control subject's white-matter voxels; this time, though, the RRMS patients' mean value was also somewhat elevated relative to controls.

Cr in PVWM and Gray Matter

Pan and Whitaker [33] found similar mean PVWM Cr values in their PPMS and their RRMS patients (Fig. 7). Although the difference between their patient groups and their normal control group was not tested statistically, it seems as

Cr in NAWM

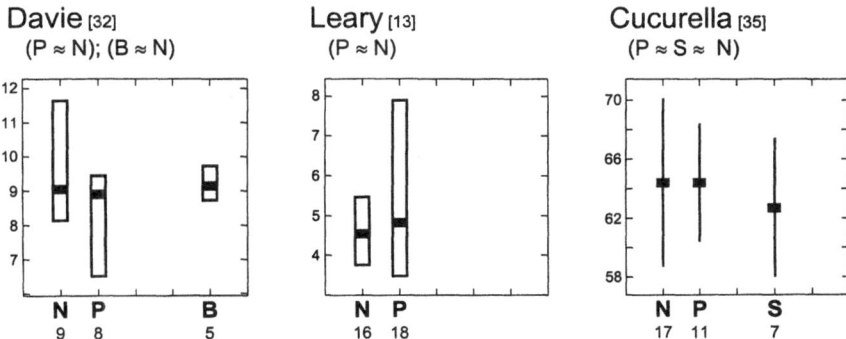

Fig. 6. Results of studies that quantified Cr resonance intensities in the NAWM of patients with primary progressive (*P*), relapsing-remitting (*R*), secondary progressive (*S*), or benign (*B*) multiple sclerosis, as well as in the normal white matter tissue of normal controls (*N*). See Fig. 2 legend for more information. Note that the normal control data in the Suhy et al. study [37] are controlled for age

though both MS groups had normal PVWM Cr levels. As for gray-matter Cr levels, Pan and Whitaker found that their PPMS patients had a lower mean-Cr-value than did their low-disability RRMS patients (who seem to be similar to their normal controls, although this also was not tested statistically). Again, however, it should be kept in mind that this abstract-based report included only four

Cr in PVWM   Cr in Grey Matter

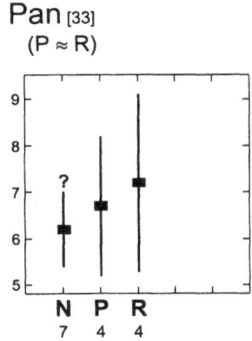   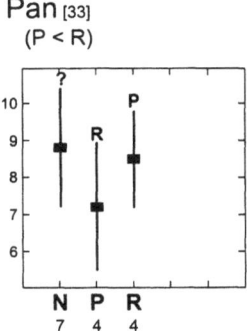

Fig. 7. Results of a study that quantified Cr resonance intensities in the PVWM and occipitoparietal gray matter of patients with primary progressive (*P*) or relapsing-remitting (*R*) multiple sclerosis, as well as in the white matter and gray matter of normal controls (*N*). ? signifies the lack of an explicit statistical comparison in the original publication. See Fig. 2 legend for more information

patients in each MS group and, thus, needs to be replicated in a larger group of patients.

Cho-Related Findings

Cho in Lesions

Three studies provided semiabsolute quantification of Cho in the lesional brain tissue of PPMS patients [32, 35, 37] (Fig. 8). All three studies were consistent with regard to PPMS: Davie et al. [32], Cucurella et al .[35], and Suhy et al. [37] all found that the average Cho values in their PPMS patients' lesions did not differ from those measured in the other patient groups' lesions or in the control subjects' white matter voxels. Unlike Davie et al. [35], however, Cucurella et al. [35] found the mean Cho value in their SPMS patients' lesion voxels to be elevated relative to their controls' data. As mentioned earlier, Cho levels measured by ^{1}H-MRS have been shown to be greatly affected by lesion activity [30] and, thus, differences in lesion activity in the patient groups in these studies may have contributed to this finding.

Cho in NAWM

The same three studies provided semiabsolute quantification of Cho in the NAWM of PPMS patients [32, 35, 37] (Fig. 9). Again, the findings in all three studies were consistent: Davie et al. [32], Cucurella et al. [35], and Suhy et al. [37] all found no significant difference between their various patient groups and their normal controls.

Cho in Lesions

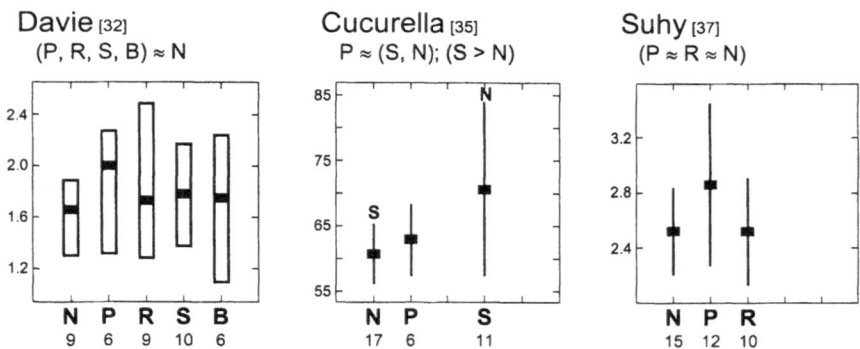

Fig. 8. Results of studies that quantified resonance intensities from choline-containing phospholipids plus other tetramethyl amines (Cho) in the lesional brain-tissue of patients with primary progressive (*P*), relapsing-remitting (*R*), secondary progressive (*S*), or benign (*B*) multiple sclerosis, as well as in the normal white matter tissue of normal controls (*N*). See Fig. 2 legend for more information

Cho in NAWM

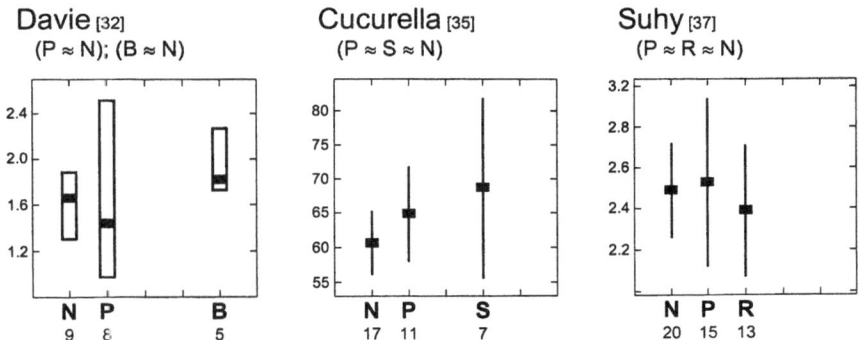

Fig. 9. Results of studies that quantified resonance intensities from Cho in the NAWM of patients with primary progressive (*P*), relapsing-remitting (*R*), secondary progressive (*S*), or benign (*B*) multiple sclerosis, as well as in the normal white matter tissue of normal controls (*N*). See Fig. 2 legend for more information

Cho in PVWM and Gray-Matter

Pan and Whitaker [33] found that their PPMS patients had a significantly lower mean Cho value than did their RRMS patients (Fig. 10). Their PPMS patients did not seem to be different from normal controls, however, suggesting that PVWM Cho was increased in the RRMS group. As for gray-matter Cho levels, Pan and

Cho in PVWM

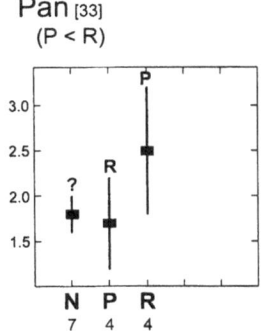

Cho in Grey Matter

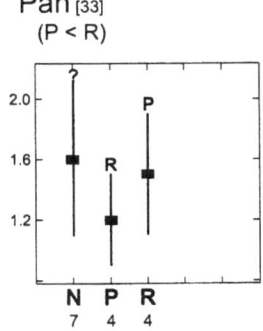

Fig. 10. Results of a study that quantified resonance intensities from Cho in the PVWM and occipitoparietal gray matter of patients with primary progressive (*P*) or relapsing-remitting (*R*) multiple sclerosis, as well as in the white matter and gray matter of normal controls (*N*). ? signifies the lack of a statistical comparison in the original publication. See Fig. 2 legend for more information

Whitaker found that their PPMS patients had a lower mean value than did their low-disability RRMS patients (who seemed to be similar to their normal controls, although this too was not tested statistically). Again, this abstract-based report included only four patients in each MS group and, thus, these findings need to be confirmed in a larger sample.

NA/Cr-Related Findings

NA/Cr in Lesions
Three studies examined NA/Cr ratios in the lesional brain-tissue of PPMS patients [34, 35, 37] (Fig. 11). All three studies were consistent with regard to PPMS: Pike et al. [34], Cucurella et al. [35], and Suhy et al. [37] all found that the average NA/Cr values in their PPMS patients' lesions did not differ from those measured in their other patient groups' lesions; furthermore, both Cucurella et al. [35] and Suhy et al. [37] found that the average NA/Cr values in their patient groups were decreased relative to their normal control subjects' white matter voxels (age-corrected values being used in the Suhy et al. study[37]). Interestingly, Pike et al. [34], who used ¹H-MRSI, found that their three patient groups had similar NA/Cr values regardless of whether they considered (1) data from only relatively-new lesions (i.e., lesions that were < 6 months old) or (2) data from these relatively new lesions combined with data from relatively old lesions (i.e., > 24 months old).

NA/Cr in NAWM
Three studies examined NA/Cr ratios in the NAWM of PPMS patients [13, 35, 37] (Fig. 12). All three had consistent findings with regard to their PPMS patients rel-

NA/Cr in Lesions

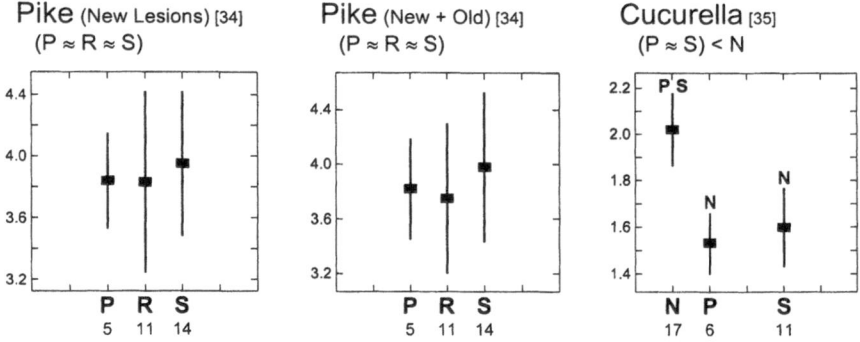

Fig. 11. Results of studies that examined the ratio of NA resonance intensities to those from Cr in the lesional brain tissue of patients with primary progressive (*P*), relapsing-remitting (*R*), or secondary progressive (*S*) multiple sclerosis, as well as in the normal white matter tissue of normal controls (*N*). See Fig. 2 legend for more information. Note that the normal control data in the Suhy et al. study [37] are controlled for age

NA/Cr in NAWM

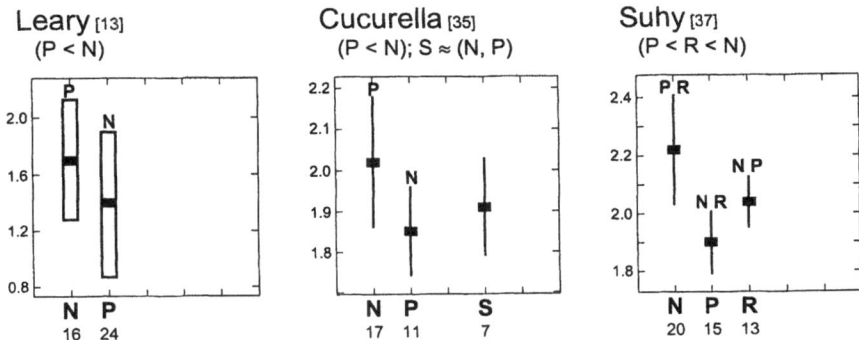

Fig. 12. Results of studies that examined the ratio of NA resonance intensities to those from Cr in the NAWM of patients with primary progressive (*P*), relapsing-remitting (*R*), or secondary progressive (*S*) multiple sclerosis, as well as in the normal white matter tissue of normal controls (*N*). See Fig. 2 legend for more information. Note that the normal control data in the Suhy et al. study [37] are controlled for age

ative to their normal controls: Leary et al. [13], Cucurella et al. [35], and Suhy et al. [37] all found lower-than-normal values in their PPMS patients. In relation to other MS groups, Cucurella et al. [35] found that their PPMS and SPMS patients had similar mean NA/Cr values and Suhy et al. [37] found that their PPMS patients had a lower mean NA/Cr value than did their RRMS patients. This last finding can be explained, however, as a difference in these patient groups' Cr values (see Fig. 6) and not in their NA values (see Fig. 3).

Leary et al. [13] also tried to look specifically at NAA/Cr in their study and, again, they found the same results as with the NA-related measure (i.e., reduced NAA/Cr values in the NAWM voxels of their PPMS patients, results not shown in Fig. 12).

NA/Cr in Non-Tissue-Specific Brain Volumes

Recently, Pelletier et al. presented two studies that used ¹H-MRSI to examine NA/Cr values in the brains of MS patients and normal controls [39, 40]. Unlike in the other studies presented above, no distinction was made between NAWM and lesional brain tissue, or between gray and white matter tissue; rather, a much larger volume of brain was examined in a non-tissue-specific manner. Indeed, this is a common practice and many ¹H-MRSI studies of MS patients have used such an approach. For example, many investigators have looked at NA/Cr ratios in large volumes of interest that have been centered over the corpus callosum [15, 17] and, more recently, others have started to look at NA/Cr ratios in the whole brain [42]. In their two studies, Pelletier et al. used 3D echo-planar ¹H-MRSI [43] to obtain NA/Cr values in either (1) a very large volume of supratentorial brain or (2) a smaller volume of brain that was centered over the corpus callosum.

As shown in Fig. 13, these two studies confirmed and complemented one another. In the first study [39], Pelletier et al. found that: (1) both their PPMS and their SPMS patients had lower mean NA/Cr ratios than their normal controls, but (2) their RRMS patients did not, on average, differ from their normal controls. Although they did not formally test the mean differences amongst their MS subgroups in this study, inspection of Fig. 13 suggests that the two progressive-MS patient groups' mean values are similar (and possibly lower than the mean value of the RRMS group). These authors also showed that measuring NA/Cr in either of these two volumes – at least the way that they did it – was effectively equivalent ($r = 0.941$, 95% confidence intervals = 0.898-0.966; mean difference between individuals' supratentorial brain and corpus callosum NA/Cr estimates = -0.062): importantly, this finding implies that volumes of interest centered on the corpus callosum provide a representative sample of the whole supratentorial brain.

In a second study [40], Pelletier and his colleagues found, again, that patients with PPMS had lower mean NA/Cr values in the supratentorial brain than did their age-matched normal controls. Interestingly, this was found in PPMS patients with either high or low lesion loads on T2-weighted MRI [mean (SD) lesion load = 10.84 (7.44) cm³, 1.41 (0.96) cm³, respectively].

Cho/Cr-Related Findings

Cho/Cr in Lesions, NAWM, and Non-Tissue-Specific Brain Volumes
Cucurella et al [35] found that their PPMS patients' mean Cho/Cr value did not differ from that of their normal controls, but that their RRMS patients' mean

NA/Cr in Brain Tissue

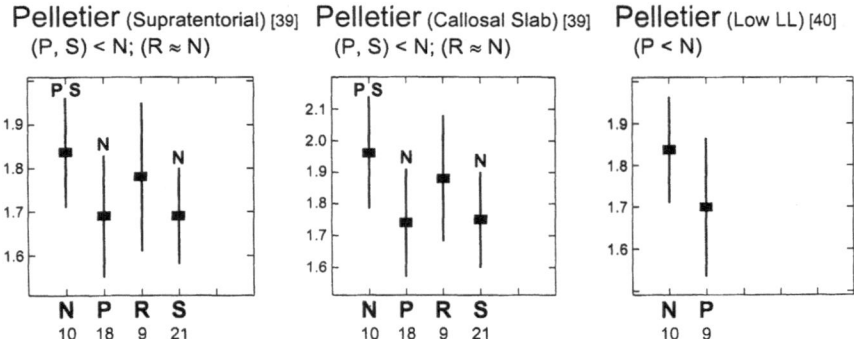

Fig.13. Results of studies that examined the ratio of NA resonance intensities to those from Cr in a very large volume of supratentorial brain, as well as in a smaller volume centered over the corpus callosum, in patients with primary progressive (*P*), relapsing-remitting (*R*), or secondary progressive (*S*) multiple sclerosis, as well as in normal controls (*N*). Note that the data in the second Pelletier et al. study [40] are all from a supratentorial brain volume and that the P patients in that study had either a high or a low lesion load (*LL*, see text). See Fig. 2 legend for more information

value was significantly increased relative to both of them (Fig. 14). It should be noted, however, that their two MS patient groups' did not differ significantly on either their mean lesional Cr values (see Fig. 5) or their mean lesional Cho values (see Fig. 8). As for NAWM, Cucurella et al. [35] found that their three groups' mean Cho/Cr values did not differ significantly. Similarly, in another study that examined Cho/Cr in PPMS patients [40] (this time in a large, non-tissue-specific volume of supratentorial brain), Pelletier et al. found that their PPMS patients with either high or low lesion loads both had mean Cho/Cr values that were similar to those in their age-matched normal controls. Unfortunately, descriptive statistics regarding these three groups' Cho/Cr values were not presented in this abstract-based report [40] and, thus, these values cannot be included here.

Correlation Between ¹H-MRS Data and Disability in PPMS

Of the eight papers that presented ¹H-MRS data from patients with PPMS, only three presented data correlating ¹H-MRS-measured metabolite values and disability as measured by patients' scores on the EDSS [7]. Davie et al. [32] found a small, but significant, negative correlation between individual patients' NAA and EDSS values ($\rho = -0.364, p < 0.05$); unfortunately, this was for all of their patients grouped together. On the other hand, both Leary et al. [13] and Suhy et al. [37] looked at this relationship specifically in PPMS patients. Leary et al. [13] reported no significant correlations between EDSS and any of the NAWM metabolite concentrations or ratios that they measured. Suhy et al. [37] also failed to find a significant correlation of EDSS with either NA or Cr values measured in the lesional tissue of their RRMS and their PPMS patients. They did, however, find that NA/Cr in the NAWM of their PPMS patients (but not of their RRMS patients)

Cho/Cr in Lesions

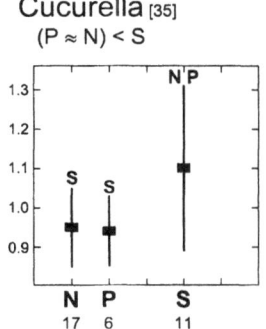

Cho/Cr in NAWM

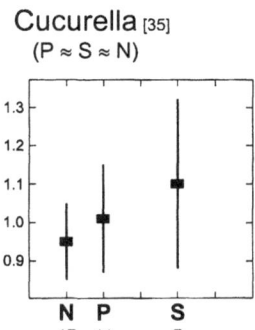

Fig. 14. Results of a study that examined the ratio of Cho resonance intensities to those from Cr in the lesional brain tissue, as well as in the NAWM, of patients with primary progressive (*P*) or secondary-progressive (*S*) multiple sclerosis, as well as in the normal white matter tissue of normal controls (*N*). See Fig. 2 legend for more information

was significantly related to these patients' EDSS scores ($r^2 = 0.67, p = 0.03, n = 12$). Nevertheless, given (1) the small sample size and (2) the fact that no significant correlation was found between lesional NA/Cr and EDSS in either of their patient groups, this last finding might not be generalizable.

Summary of PPMS Findings

Table 3 summarizes most of the ^{1}H-MRS and ^{1}H-MRSI findings in the PPMS patients reviewed above. As can be seen therein, despite (1) the relatively low sample sizes, (2) the cross-study differences in patients' clinical and demographic characteristics, and (3) the cross-study differences in imaging and metabolite quantification techniques used, the studies reviewed here show, for the most part, remarkable consistency.

NA and NA/Cr Values
There is complete agreement that, as a group, PPMS patients have reduced NA and NA/Cr values relative to those found in the white matter of normal controls: this holds true for (1) voxels that are filled with NAWM [13, 32, 35, 37] and (2) voxels that are filled with lesional brain-tissue [32, 34, 35, 37], as well as for (3) larger volumes of non-tissue-specific brain [39, 40]. There is also complete agreement that PPMS patients do not differ from either RRMS or SPMS patients in terms of their mean within-lesional NA and NA/Cr values [34, 35, 37]. There is also almost complete agreement that mean NAWM NA and NA/Cr values are similar in PPMS, RRMS, and SPMS patients [35, 37] – the only incongruous finding being that of Suhy et al. [37], who found that, on average, NA/Cr values were somewhat less reduced in the NAWM of their RRMS patients (see Fig. 12). This was due to a difference in Cr, however, and not to a difference in NA (see below). In summary, these findings suggest that there is, indeed, ^{1}H-MRS evidence of neuronal disturbance (at least as reflected in NA-related measures) in the brains of PPMS patients, but that this disturbance is equivalent to that found in RRMS and SPMS patients.

Cho and Cho/Cr Values
There is also complete agreement that, on average, Cho and Cho/Cr values in PPMS patients do not differ from those measured in the white matter of normal controls: this holds true for voxels that are filled either with NAWM [32, 35, 37], lesional brain-tissue [32, 35, 37], or non-tissue-specific brain [40]. There is also agreement that PPMS patients do not differ from either RRMS or SPMS patients in terms of (1) their mean within-lesion Cho values [35, 37], or (2) their mean NAWM Cho and Cho/Cr values [35, 37]. One study [35] did, however, find that SPMS patients had higher lesional Cho/Cr values than did PPMS patients (even though these same patients did not differ statistically in either their Cho or their Cr values). Unfortunately, no attempt was made in that study to correlate the age of the individuals' lesions with their Cho/Cr values (an analysis that might have

Table 3. Table summarizing the statistically-significant ¹H-MRS findings in the lesional, normal-appearing white matter (NAWM), and non-tissue-specific brain of patients with primary progressive multiple sclerosis (PP) versus those with relapsing-remitting (RR) or secondary-progressive (SP) multiple sclerosis, as well as in PP patients versus the white matter tissue of normal controls (NC).

Measure	Statistically-significant findings			Study
	PP vs RR	PP vs SP	PP vs NC	
Cerebrospinal fluid	≈	•	↓ᵃ	Nicoli et al. [31]
NA in lesions	•	•	↓	Davie et al. [32]
	•	ª	↓	Cucurella et al. [35]
	≈	•	↓	Suhy et al. [37]
NA in NAWM	•	•	↓	Davie et al. [32]
	•	•	↓ᵇ	Leary et al. [13]
	•	ª	↓	Cucurella et al. [35]
	≈	•	↓	Suhy et al. [37]
Cr in lesions	•	•	≈	Davie et al. [32]
	•	•	•	Cucurella et al. [35]
	↑	•	↑	Suhy et al. [37]
Cr in NAWM	•	•	≈	Davie et al. [32]
	•	•	≈	Leary et al. [13]
	•	≈	≈	Cucurella et al. [35]
	↑	•	↑	Suhy et al. [37]
Cho in lesions	•	•	ª	Davie et al. [32]
	•	≈	≈	Cucurella et al. [35]
	≈	•	≈	Suhy et al. [37]
Cho in NAWM	•	•	ª	Davie et al. [32]
	•	≈	≈	Cucurella et al. [35]
	≈	•	≈	Suhy et al. [37]
NA/Cr in lesions	≈ᶜ	≈ᶜ	•	Pike et al. [34]
	•	≈	↓	Cucurella et al. [35]
	≈	•	↓	Suhy et al. [37]
NA/Cr in NAWM	•	•	↓ᵇ	Leary et al. [13]
	•	≈	↓	Cucurella et al. [35]
	↓ᵈ	•	↓	Suhy et al. [37]
NA/Cr in brain	•	•	↓ᵉ	Pelletier et al. [39]
	•	•	↓ᶠ	Pelletier et al. [40]
Cho/Cr in lesions	•	↓ᵍ	≈	Cucurella et al. [35]
Cho/Cr in NAWM	•	≈	≈	Cucurella et al. [35]
Cho/Cr in brain	•	•	≈ʰ	Pelletier et al. [40]

• difference not tested; ≈ no significant difference; ↓ PP significantly decreased; ↑ PP significantly increased; *NA*, N-acetyl groups; *Cr*, creatine plus phosphocreatine; *Cho*, choline-containing phospholipids plus other tetramethyl amines

ª Patients were compared with diseased controls and changes were found in a number of CSF metabolites

ᵇ Similar results were found for N-acetyl aspartate (i.e., NAA)

ᶜ Similar results were found for new lesions (i.e., < 6 months old) and for all lesions combined

ᵈ These results are due to a difference in Cr, not NA

ᵉ Similar results were found in a very large volume of supratentorial brain and in a smaller volume of brain that was centered over the corpus callosum

ᶠ Similar results were found in patients with either high or low lesion loads (see text)

ᵍ The authors of this study questioned the meaning of this particular set of findings

ʰ The authors did not provide any descriptive statistics but they did state that similar results were found in both their high- and low-lesion load subgroups

helped to explain those findings). Thus, in summary, it seems that there is little, or no, ^{1}H-MRS evidence of significant myelin breakdown in the brains of the PPMS patients studied thus far – either as compared to normal controls or as compared to patients with RRMS or SPMS. Of course, the lesions that were studied in all of these patients were all relatively chronic and these findings might not hold true if more acute lesions were studied.

Cr Values

Of the studies that quantified Cr values in patients with PPMS, all but one found that Cr was normal in these patients' lesions [32, 35] as well as in their NAWM [13, 32, 35]. One study, however, found that Cr was elevated in both the lesional and the NAWM tissue of PPMS patients, both with respect to such tissue in RRMS patients and to the white matter of normal controls [37]. It is unclear, however, what is responsible for these conflicting findings; for example, differences in metabolite quantification (see section above on Cr-related findings) or differences in lesion "age" (which was not specified in the conflicting study but has been shown to be related to Cr values in MS patients, see, e.g., [25]).

Overall Conclusions

As we have seen, patients with PPMS are as disabled as those with the SP form of the disease. Furthermore, as we have reviewed above, ^{1}H-MRS and ^{1}H-MRSI changes are, indeed, found in PPMS. Nevertheless, as is the case with PPMS patients' lesion loads and their spinal cord cross-sectional areas, these spectroscopy-related changes are not in step with their observed disabilities. Thus, examining these patients with ^{1}H-MRS and ^{1}H-MRSI does not seem to be have helped us in resolving the paradox regarding the disparity between the disability seen in these patients and their findings on quantitative neuroimaging. It is possible, however, that the answer to this riddle is simply beyond the methodologies used thus far. Indeed, it may turn out that an extension (e.g., the simultaneous, high-resolution, multimodel consideration of the entire neuraxis) of the measures reviewed herein – as well as those of other sophisticated imaging modalities (e.g., measures of magnetization transfer, atrophy, diffusion, and diffusion anisotropy) – will be required in order to describe fully a pathology that is discriminatively characteristic of PPMS. Fortunately, with the advances that are continually being made in the neuroimaging technologies, this may become feasible in even the not-too-distant future.

References

1. Lublin FD, Reingold SC (1996) Defining the clinical course of multiple sclerosis: results of an international survey. National Multiple Sclerosis Society (USA) Advisory Committee on Clinical Trials of New Agents in Multiple Sclerosis. Neurology 46:907-911

2. Thompson AJ, Montalban X, Barkhof F et al (2000) Diagnostic criteria for primary progressive multiple sclerosis: a position paper. Ann Neurol 47:831-835
3. Li DK, Zhao G, Paty DW (2000) T2 hyperintensities: findings and significance. Neuroimaging Clin N Am 10:717-738
4. Allen IV, McKeown SR (1979) A histological, histochemical and biochemical study of the macroscopically normal white matter in multiple sclerosis. J Neurol Sci 41:81-91
5. Allen IV, Glover G, Anderson R (1981) Abnormalities in the macroscopically normal white matter in cases of mild or spinal multiple sclerosis (MS). Acta Neuropathol Suppl (Berl) 7:176-178
6. Trapp BD, Peterson J, Ransohoff RM et al (1998) Axonal transection in the lesions of multiple sclerosis. N Engl J Med 338:278-285
7. Kurtzke JF (1983) Rating neurologic impairment in multiple sclerosis: an expanded disability status scale (EDSS). Neurology 33:1444-1452
8. Thompson AJ, Kermode AG, MacManus DG et al (1990) Patterns of disease activity in multiple sclerosis: clinical and magnetic resonance imaging study. Br Med J 300:631-634
9. Stevenson VL, Miller DH, Rovaris M et al (1999) Primary and transitional progressive MS: a clinical and MRI cross-sectional study. Neurology 52:839-845
10. Thompson AJ, Kermode AG, MacManus DG et al (1989) Pathogenesis of progressive multiple sclerosis. Lancet 1:1322-1323
11. Thompson AJ, Kermode AG, Wicks D et al (1991) Major differences in the dynamics of primary and secondary progressive multiple sclerosis. Ann Neurol 29:53-62
12. Lycklama à Nijeholt GJ, van Walderveen MA, Castelijns JA et al (1998) Brain and spinal cord abnormalities in multiple sclerosis. Correlation between MRI parameters, clinical subtypes and symptoms. Brain 121:687-697
13. Leary SM, Davie CA, Parker GJ et al (1999) ^{1}H magnetic resonance spectroscopy of normal appearing white matter in primary progressive multiple sclerosis. J Neurol 246:1023-1026
14. Thompson AJ, Polman CH, Miller DH et al (1997) Primary progressive multiple sclerosis. Brain 120:1085-1096
15. Arnold DL, De Stefano N, Narayanan S, Matthews PM (2000) Proton MR spectroscopy in multiple sclerosis. Neuroimaging Clin N Am 10:789-798
16. Ross B, Bluml S (2001) Magnetic resonance spectroscopy of the human brain. Anat Rec (New Anat) 265:54-84
17. De Stefano N, Narayanan S, Francis GS et al (2001) Evidence of axonal damage in the early stages of multiple sclerosis and its relevance to disability. Arch Neurol 58:65-70
18. Narayanan S, De Stefano N, Francis GS et al (2001) Axonal metabolic recovery in multiple sclerosis patients treated with interferon β-1b. J Neurol 248:979-986
19. Provencher SW (1993) Estimation of metabolite concentrations from localized in vivo proton NMR spectra. Magn Reson Med 30:672-679
20. Christiansen P, Henriksen O, Stubgaard M et al (1993) In vivo quantification of brain metabolites by ^{1}H-MRS using water as an internal standard. Magn Reson Imaging 11:107-118
21. Pan JW, Twieg DB, Hetherington HP (1998) Quantitative spectroscopic imaging of the human brain. Magn Reson Med 40:363-369
22. Urenjak J, Williams SR, Gadian DG, Noble M (1993) Proton nuclear magnetic resonance spectroscopy unambiguously identifies different neural cell types. J Neurosci 13:981-989
23. Chang L, Ernst T, Osborn D et al (1998) Proton spectroscopy in myotonic dystrophy: correlations with CTG repeats. Arch Neurol 55:305-311
24. De Stefano N, Matthews PM, Antel JP et al (1995) Chemical pathology of acute demyelinating lesions and its correlation with disability. Ann Neurol 38:901-909
25. Helms G, Stawiarz L, Kivisakk P, Link H (2000) Regression analysis of metabolite concentrations estimated from localized proton MR spectra of active and chronic multiple sclerosis lesions. Magn Reson Med 43:102-110

26. Sarchielli P, Presciutti O, Pelliccioli GP et al (1999) Absolute quantification of brain metabolites by proton magnetic resonance spectroscopy in normal-appearing white matter of multiple sclerosis patients. Brain 122:513-521

27. Simmons ML, Frondoza CG, Coyle JT (1991) Immunocytochemical localization of N-acetyl-aspartate with monoclonal antibodies. Neuroscience 45:37-45

28. Arnold DL, Matthews PM, Francis G, Antel J (1990) Proton magnetic resonance spectroscopy of human brain in vivo in the evaluation of multiple sclerosis: assessment of the load of disease. Magn Reson Med 14:154-159

29. Bitsch A, Bruhn H, Vougioukas V et al (1999) Inflammatory CNS demyelination: histopathologic correlation with in vivo quantitative proton MR spectroscopy. AJNR Am J Neuroradiol 20:1619-1627

30. Arnold DL, Matthews PM, Francis GS et al (1992) Proton magnetic resonance spectroscopic imaging for metabolic characterization of demyelinating plaques. Ann Neurol 31:235-241

31. Nicoli F, Vion-Dury J, Confort-Gouny S et al (1996) Cerebrospinal fluid metabolic profiles in multiple sclerosis and degenerative dementias obtained by high resolution proton magnetic resonance spectroscopy. C R Acad Sci III 319:623-631

32. Davie CA, Barker GJ, Thompson AJ et al (1997) ^{1}H magnetic resonance spectroscopy of chronic cerebral white matter lesions and normal appearing white matter in multiple sclerosis. J Neurol Neurosurg Psychiatry 63:736-742

33. Pan JW, Whitaker JN (1998) Quantitation of ^{1}H metabolites in subtypes of multiple sclerosis by spectroscopic imaging at 4.1 T [abstract]. Proc Int Soc Magn Reson Med 1:428

34. Pike GB, de Stefano N, Narayanan S et al (1999) Combined magnetization transfer and proton spectroscopic imaging in the assessment of pathologic brain lesions in multiple sclerosis. AJNR Am J Neuroradiol 20:829-837

35. Cucurella MG, Rovira A, Rio J et al (2000) Proton magnetic resonance spectroscopy in primary and secondary progressive multiple sclerosis. NMR Biomed 13:57-63

36. Pan JW, Krupp LB, Elkins L, Coyle PK (2000) Cognitive dysfunction lateralizes with NAA in multiple sclerosis [abstract]. Proc Intl Soc Magn Reson Med 1:296

37. Suhy J, Rooney WD, Goodkin DE et al (2000) ^{1}H MRSI comparison of white matter and lesions in primary progressive and relapsing-remitting MS. Mult Scler 6:148-155

38. Oh J, Pelletier D, Nelson SJ (2001) Proton magnetic resonance spectroscopy in assessing axonal loss in the corpus callosum related with volume of regional T_1 lesion load in multiple sclerosis [abstract]. Proc Int Soc Mag Reson Med 2:471

39. Pelletier D, Grenier D, Lu Y et al (2001) Regional comparison of axonal damage in multiple sclerosis using whole supratentorial brain 3D spectroscopy imaging [abstract]. Proc Int Soc Magn Reson Med 2:985

40. Pelletier D, Grenier D, Antel JP et al (2001) MRI lesion volume heterogeneity in primary progressive multiple sclerosis: an assessment of axonal damage and brain atrophy measurement [abstract]. Neurology 56:A380

41. Viala K, Stievenart JL, Cabanis EA et al (2001) Study with localized proton magnetic resonance spectroscopy of 31 multiple sclerosis lesions: correlations with clinical and MRI features (in French). Rev Neurol (Paris) 157:35-44

42. Gonen O, Catalaa I, Babb JS et al (2000) Total brain N-acetylaspartate: a new measure of disease load in MS. Neurology 54:15-19

43. Posse S, DeCarli C, Le Bihan D (1994) Three-dimensional echo-planar MR spectroscopic imaging at short echo times in the human brain. Radiology 192:733-738

44. Van den Boogaart A, Vanhamme L (1997) MRUI Manual v. 96.3. A User's Guide to the Magnetic Resonance User Interface software package. Delft Technische Universiteit Press, Delft

Chapter 10

Functional Magnetic Resonance Imaging

M. FILIPPI, M.A. ROCCA

Introduction

In multiple sclerosis (MS), the clinical manifestations and the patterns of disease evolution are highly variable and correlate only weakly with findings on conventional magnetic resonance imaging (MRI) scans of the brain [1-3]. During the last few years, significant effort has been devoted to the definition of the factors contributing to this clinical/MRI discrepancy with the ultimate goal of achieving a better understanding of the mechanisms leading to irreversible disability in MS [4].

Although numerous studies have shown the importance of several factors in determining MS-related disability [5-11], including the severity of intrinsic lesion damage, the location of lesion, the extent and nature of microscopic changes in the normal-appearing white matter (NAWM), and the severity of spinal cord damage, the strength of the correlation between disability and MRI findings is still suboptimal in patients with MS [12]. The variable presence and efficacy of "reparative" mechanisms with the potential to limit the functional impact of tissue damage in MS might yet prove to be an additional factor that reduces the magnitude of the relationship between MRI measures of pathology and clinical measures of disability. Among these factors, adaptive cortical reorganization following tissue damage is likely to have an important role. This is why functional MRI (fMRI) holds substantial promise to improve our understanding of the pathophysiology of MS.

Basic Principles of fMRI

FMRI is a relatively new MRI technique that is being widely used to study the neuronal mechanisms of central nervous system (CNS) functioning, and which can be used to define abnormal patterns of brain activations arising from disease. The signal changes seen during fMRI studies depend on the blood-oxygenation-level-dependent (BOLD) mechanism, which in turn involves changes of the transverse magnetization relaxation time – either $T2^*$, in a gradient echo sequence, or $T2$, in a spin echo sequence. These changes are attributable to differences in deoxyhemoglobin consequent upon variations in neuronal activity [13]. The correlation between local deoxyhemoglobin levels and neuronal activity is thought to result from changes in oxygen extraction, cerebral blood flow (CBF), and cerebral blood volume (CBV) [13], all of which change with neuronal activity [14-17]. Activation of a given brain area produces an increase in the neuronal and glial metabolism, accompanied by an increase in the regional CBF of that area. Although it has not yet been proven for all the stimuli, there is evidence that, initially, the oxygenation level of the blood drops slightly ("early response" or "initial dip") [15]. This event is followed by an increase in both blood flow and oxygen concentration ("late" response) (Fig. 1). As a consequence, three effects can contribute to the fMRI signal changes: (1) an increase in the blood flow velocity, (2) an increase in the blood volume flow rate, and (3) changes in the blood oxygenation level. When fast MRI methods are used, the contribution of the last factor is maximized [17, 18].

In comparison with other functional techniques, such as positron emission tomography (PET), fMRI is completely noninvasive, less expensive, and gives better spatial resolution. The higher spatial resolution allows better definition of anatomical areas involved in task performance. In addition, registration of fMR with structural MRI is easier, since both can be acquired in the same scanning session.

FMRI in MS

FMRI has been applied to the study of the visual and motor system functioning of patients with relapsing-remitting and secondary progressive MS or with clinically isolated syndromes suggestive of MS [19-25].

In a preliminary study examining the visual system [19], MS patients with unilateral optic neuritis (ON) had a smaller activation of the visual cortex after stim-

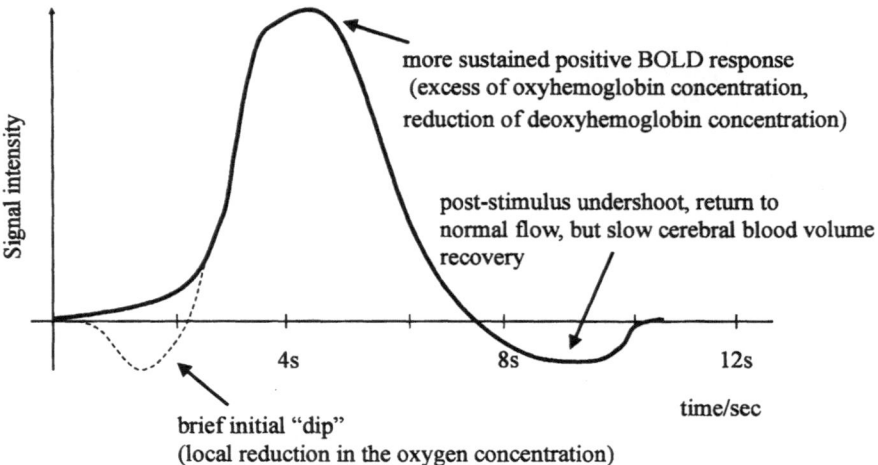

Fig. 1. Schematic of the course of the blood-oxygenation-level-dependent (BOLD) response to an increase in neuronal activity. The *dotted line* indicates that the brief initial dip of the BOLD response has not been proved definitively

ulation of the affected and the unaffected eyes than did healthy subjects. On average, recovered patients showed greater visual cortex activation than did nonrecovered patients, although activation in the former group was reduced compared to that found in healthy individuals. More recently, Werring et al. [20] conducted a similar study on patients who had recovered from a single episode of acute unilateral ON. While in controls visual stimulation activated only the primary visual cortex, in patients extensive activations of the claustrum, lateral temporal and posterior parietal cortices, and thalamus were also found when the clinically affected eye was studied. Stimulation of the clinically unaffected eye activated the visual cortex and the right insula-claustrum only. In addition, the volume of the extraoccipital activation in patients with ON was found to correlate strongly with the latency of the visual evoked potential. Since all the activated extraoccipital areas have been shown to be part of a complex network responsible for multimodal integration [26], the findings of this study fit with the notion that a functional reorganization of the cerebral response might represent an adaptive response to a persistently abnormal visual input.

FMRI has also been used to evaluate motor system functioning in clinically stable MS patients and in MS patients during recovery after an acute relapse. Clanet et al. [21] obtained fMRI from eight patients with clinically definite MS presenting with acute or chronic motor deficits of the upper limb. In normal controls, the performance of a simple motor task elicited a constant activation of the contralateral primary sensorimotor cortex (SMC) and, sometimes, a smaller activation of the ipsilateral primary motor cortex and the supplementary motor area (SMA). The cerebellum was also activated bilaterally, but the activation was more evident ipsilaterally to the tested limb. In MS patients able to perform the task, the contralateral primary motor cortex was always activated, whereas no activation was detected in those patients unable to perform the task. Compared to normal controls, MS patients with partial motor weakness showed larger activations of the ipsilateral and contralateral areas involved in motor execution and programming. In this study [21], two patients were also evaluated serially during the recovery after an acute paralysis of the upper extremities. In one of these patients, initially unable to perform the task, no activation was observed. However, when the "normal" hand was used to perform the task, the primary motor cortex was activated bilaterally. During clinical recovery of the affected hand, a bilateral activation of the primary motor cortex with a transient significant increase of the activated area was observed.

These observations have been confirmed and extended by Lee et al. [22], who used fMRI to characterize the site and volume of motor cortex activations during flexion-extension of the last four fingers in 12 clinically stable patients with relapsing-remitting and secondary progressive MS. They found greater SMA activation in MS patients than in controls, reduced activation of the contralateral SMC in patients with more severe functional impairment, and increased ipsilateral SMC activation with increasing lesion load in the contralateral hemisphere. They also described a posterior shift of the center of activation of the contralateral SMC in patients compared to controls. The magnitude of the SMC posterior shift increased with increasing T2-weighted MRI lesion loads. These observations demonstrate that cortical recruitment for simple finger movements can change both quantitatively and qualitatively in the SMC areas of MS patients, suggesting that cortical reorganization can contribute to functional recovery.

Recent postmortem [27, 28] and in vivo quantitative MRI [5, 6, 7, 10, 29-32] studies have shown that irreversible axonal damage forms a major component of the pathology of active and chronic lesions as well as of NAWM at all phases of the disease. Despite this, quite a large number of patients with MS, at least during a certain period of their disease course, experience relapses and accumulation of MRI lesion burden without being left with any major residual neurological deficits. In the case of axonal loss, many of the factors with the potential to limit the clinical impact of damaging MS pathology [33-35], including resolution of acute inflammation, redistribution of voltage-gated sodium channels, and recovery from sublethal axonal injury, are all likely to have a limited role. To better understand whether adaptive cortical reorganization has a role in limiting the impact of irreversible tissue loss, a few recent studies have investigated the brain patterns of cortical activation during the performance of simple motor tasks in MS patients with unimpaired motor function [23-25]. Reddy et al. [23] obtained MR spectroscopy (MRS) and fMRI studies from nine MS patients who had unimpaired motor or sensory hand function. They found that activation of the ipsilateral SMC cortex with simple hand movements was increased by a mean of five-fold relative to normal controls, and that the extent of this increase correlated strongly with decreasing levels of brain N-acetylaspartate (NAA), which is considered a marker of axonal density and functioning [36]. In another paper [24], Reddy et al. followed with serial MRS and fMRI a single MS patient with a new large demyelinating lesion in the corticospinal tract after the onset of acute hemiparesis. They showed that clinical recovery preceded complete normalization of NAA levels and was accompanied by relative increases of ipsilateral primary SMC and SMA activations. This suggests that this altered pattern of recruitment of elements of the cortical motor network might have contributed to maintaining normal levels of function despite injury to the corticospinal tract. The correlation of MRS findings and fMRI responses in these two studies also suggests that dynamic reorganization of the motor cortex can occur in response to axonal injury associated with MS relapses, and that cortical reorganization might limit the functional consequences of irreversible tissue loss in MS. These observations have been extended by Rocca et al. [25], who used fMRI and a general search method to assess the pattern of brain activations associated with a simple motor task in 14 nondisabled patients with relapsing-remitting MS. In this study, the extent of the correlation between fMRI changes with T2 lesion volume and severity of MS pathology in lesions and NAWM, measured using magnetization transfer (MT) and diffusion tensor (DT) MRI, were also investigated. Compared to controls, MS patients showed increased activation in the contralateral primary SMC, bilaterally in the SMA, bilaterally in the cingulate motor area, in the contralateral ascending bank of the sylvian fissure, and in the contralateral intraparietal sulcus (Fig. 2). Several strong correlations were found between the extent of fMRI activations and several MT and DT MRI measures of structural brain damage (Fig. 2). This study showed that cortical activation occurs over a rather distributed sensorimotor network in nondisabled relapsing-remitting MS and gave additional evidence that increased recruitment of this cortical network contributes to the limitation of the functional impact of MS damage associated with macroscopic lesions and NAWM changes.

Although the mechanisms leading to adaptive cortical changes in MS are not known, it is likely that short-term changes can be mediated by recruitment of parallel existing pathways by disinhibition, whereas long-term changes might arise from new synapse formation and axonal sprouting [37-41]. Nevertheless, whatever the mechanisms leading to cortical reorganization in MS, all the above-mentioned studies [19-25] consistently showed that compensatory cortical adaptive responses do occur in patients with relapsing-remitting and secondary progressive MS. This has three major implications. First, intersubject variability in cortical reorganization might yet be an additional factor accounting for the limited relationship between conventional MRI measures of lesion burden and clinical disability. Second, these results suggest that therapies directed towards promoting cortical reorganization in response to brain injury could enhance functional recovery from MS injury. Third, these findings raise the question of whether the transition from relapsing-remitting to secondary progressive MS could be explained, at least partially, by a progressive failure of cortical adaptation mechanisms.

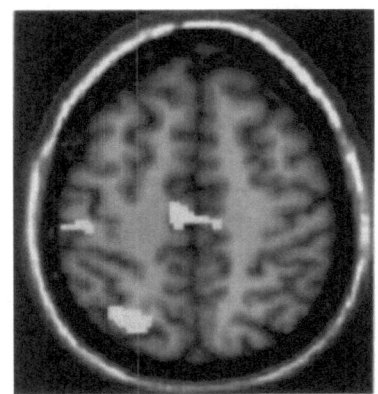

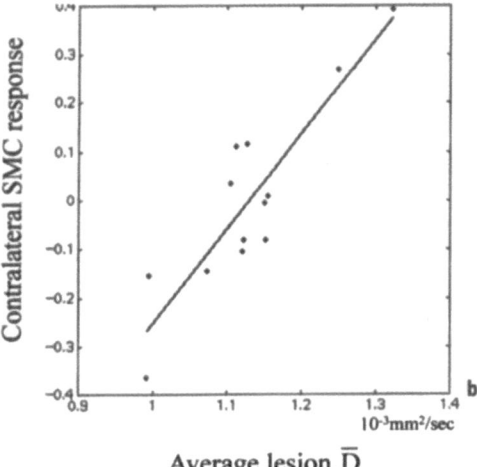

Average lesion $\bar{D}$
r = 0.88, p<0.001

Fig. 2a, b. Relative cortical activations in nondisabled relapsing-remitting MS patients during a simple motor task with the right hand in comparison to healthy volunteers. **a** Contralateral primary sensorimotor cortex (SMC), ipsi- and contralateral supplementary motor areas, and contralateral intraparietal sulcus. **b** Correlations between contralateral SMC response and average lesion mean diffusivity ($\bar{D}$)

FMRI in Patients with Primary Progressive MS

Patients with primary progressive MS (PPMS) represent 10%-15% of patients with MS and are characterized by progressive accumulation of disability from the onset of the disease [42]. This is in contrast with the small amount of lesions visible on conventional MRI scans of the brain and cord [8, 43-46]. However, MT and DT MRI as well as MRS studies have shown diffuse changes in the NAWM of the brain and cervical cord of these patients, which have been found to be correlated with disability accumulation [2, 7, 9, 10, 47-50]. Work with DT MRI has also detected widespread cortical gray matter pathology in these patients [51].

As yet, the role of brain plasticity in limiting the functional consequences of structural damage in PPMS patients has not been investigated. Understanding to which extent cortical reorganization occurs in PPMS and whether it has an adaptive role might be rewarding in terms of a better understanding of the pathophysiology of progressive disability in MS and in terms of planning treatment strategies for the affected patients. To this end, we recently performed three studies in patients with PPMS using fMRI and a general search method. The results of these studies are reviewed and discussed below.

Study 1

We assessed the patterns of brain activations following simple and complex motor tasks in 30 right-handed patients with PPMS and variable degrees of motor impairment and compared them with those from 15 right-handed sex- and age-matched controls. We found significant cortical activation changes during both simple and complex motor tasks in PPMS patients in comparison with healthy controls. PPMS patients showed a different pattern of cortical activations according to their clinical impairment. During the performance of a simple motor task with clinically unaffected limbs, PPMS patients had larger and more significant activations of the contralateral SMA, the upper bank of the sylvian fissure (SII) bilaterally, and everal regions of the frontal (bilateral middle frontal gyrus and contralateral inferior frontal gyrus) and temporal lobes (ipsilateral insula and superior temporal gyrus, bilaterally) in comparison with healthy volunteers (Fig. 3). These findings indicate a marked cortical reorganization taking place in brain regions involved in different phases of movement planning and execution. Interestingly, the observed pattern of cortical activations involves a widespread network usually considered to function in motor, sensory, and multimodal integration processing [26]. This is consistent with the notion that motor planning and execution is based on a distributed, interacting cortical network which extends well beyond "classical" motor areas [26]. During the performance of a simple task with an affected limb, PPMS patients showed increased activations of the ipsilateral cingulate motor area and the ipsilateral postcentral gyrus. Since cingulate motor area activation in healthy subjects has been related to learning of new motor tasks and is also thought to reflect task difficulty [52-54], a possible explanation for the increased cingulate motor area activity found in PPMS patients

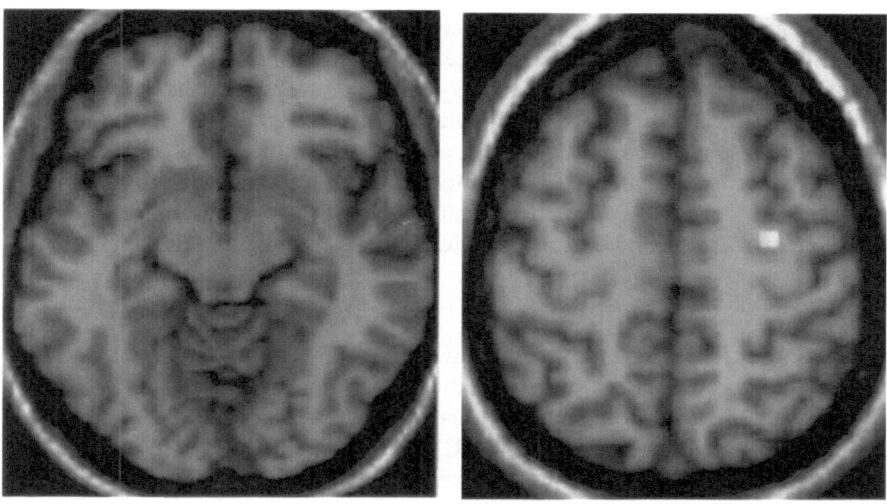

a   b

Fig. 3a, b. Relative cortical activations in right-handed patients with primary progressive MS during the performance of a simple motor task with their clinically unimpaired, right hand. **a** Ipsilateral and contralateral superior temporal gyrus. **b** Ipsilateral middle frontal gyrus

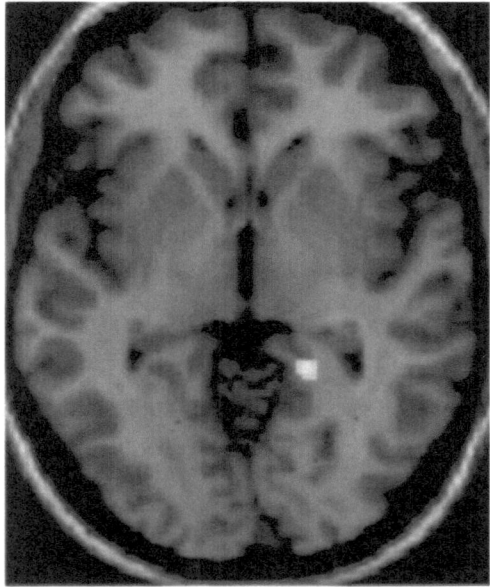

Fig. 4. Relative cortical activations of a region located in the visual cortex in right-handed patients with primary progressive MS during the performance of a complex motor task

might be that the patients tended to perceive the simple experimental task as a sort of a novel task, which, in consequence, needed to be "relearned". Finally, during the execution of a more complex task, PPMS patients showed increased activations of the ipsilateral thalamus, the middle frontal gyrus, bilaterally, and several other sensory regions, including an ipsilateral area located in the visual cortex (Fig. 4). Visual-sensory interactions are known to occur in humans [55] and, again, they might be enhanced in PPMS patients in an attempt to compensate for the functional impairment secondary to subcortical white matter damage.

Study 2

To assess whether cortical reorganization contributes to functional recovery after tissue damage in PPMS, we investigated whether the extent of brain activations during simple hand movements was correlated to lesion burden as seen on T2-weighted MRI scans, and MT ratio (MTR) and average diffusivity ($\bar{D}$) of brain T2-visible lesions, brain NAWM, and cervical cord tissue in 26 PPMS patients with fully normal motor function of the right upper limb. T2 lesion volume reflects the extent of overall MS macroscopic pathology, whereas MTR and $\bar{D}$ also provide quantitative information about tissue integrity at a microscopic level. A low MTR indicates a reduced exchange of magnetization between the protons in the brain tissue and the surrounding water protons, and in a post-mortem study [56] it was found to be strongly associated with the degree of myelin and axon loss. $\bar{D}$ is a measure of the average water molecular motion independent of any tissue directionality and is affected by cellular size and integrity [57]. We reasoned that if cortical adaptive responses have the potential to limit the accumulation of disability in patients with PPMS after tissue injury, the extent of such changes should be greater with increasing volumes of T2-visible lesions and the severity of intrinsic tissue damage in brain T2-visible lesions, brain NAWM, and cervical cord damage. Consistently with this hypothesis, we found strong correlations between the extent of the fMRI activations of several sensorimotor areas and several MR measures of structural damage of the brain and the cervical cord (Fig. 5). These findings suggest that not only brain, but also cord pathology can induce cortical changes with the potential to limit the functional impact of the disease.

Study 3

To investigate whether lesion location influences the brain pattern of cortical activations in PPMS patients, we assessed, in 15 PPMS patients with a right hemiparesis, whether the brain pattern of cortical activations was different in patients with lesions along the pyramidal tracts contralateral to the task performance compared to those without such lesions. Compared to those with lesions in the pyramidal tract, the eight PPMS patients without lesions showed relatively larger and more significant activations of the ipsilateral middle frontal gyrus. They also showed a posterior shift of the activation of the contralateral primary SMC. Compared to those without lesions in the pyramidal tract, the seven PPMS patients with lesions had relatively larger and more significant activation of the

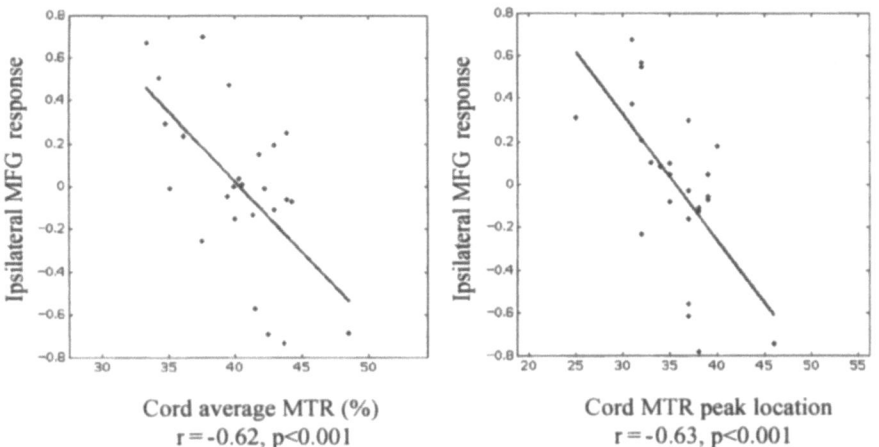

Fig. 5. Correlation between relative activation in the ipsilateral middle frontal gyrus (MFG) and average magnetization transfer ratio (MTR) (**a**) and MTR histogram peak location (**b**) of the cervical cord in patients with primary progressive MS

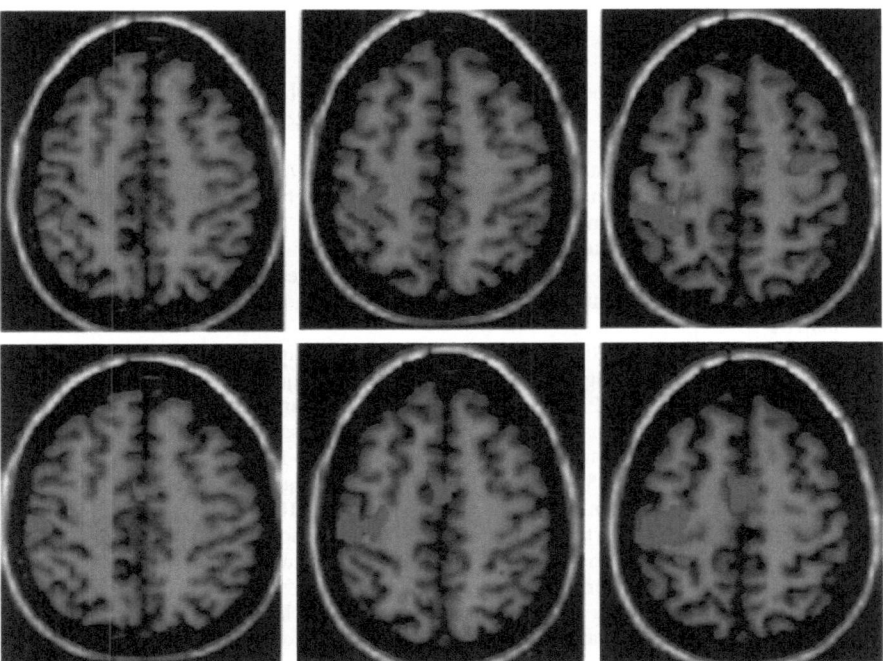

Fig. 6. Brain patterns of cortical activations following simple right hand movements in right-handed patients with primary progressive MS with a right-sided hemiparesis and with (*upper row*) or without (*lower row*) lesions in the contralateral pyramidal tract of the upper limb, according to their lesion location. See text for additional details

SMA, bilaterally (Fig. 6). These findings suggest that not only the overall burden of the disease, but also individual lesions located in critical areas can induce short- and long-distance cortical changes.

Conclusions

FMRI has the potential to provide important information about cortical reorganization following MS tissue damage which should improve our understanding of the factors associated with the progressive accumulation of irreversible disability in MS. Our studies demonstrated that cortical functional changes do also occur in patients with PPMS, and involve a widespread network usually regarded as functioning in motor, sensory, and multimodal integration processing. Although the role of cortical reorganization in limiting the functional impact of MS structural damage is still not definitively proved, our results agree with previous work [19-25] and support the concept that cortical adaptive responses may have an important role in compensating for tissue damage in MS. They also suggest that the rate of accumulation of disability in MS may be a function not only of tissue loss, but also of progressive failure of adaptive capacity of the cortex.

References

1. Filippi M, Paty DW, Kappos L et al (1995) Correlations between changes in disability and T2-weighted brain MRI activity in multiple sclerosis: a follow-up study. Neurology 45:255-260
2. Lycklama à Nijeholt GJ, van Walderveen MA, Castelijns JA et al (1998) Brain and spinal cord abnormalities in multiple sclerosis. Correlation between MRI parameters, clinical subtypes and symptoms. Brain 121:687-697
3. Kappos L, Moeri D, Radue EW et al (1999) Predictive value of gadolinium-enhanced magnetic resonance imaging for relapse rate and changes in disability or impairment in multiple sclerosis: a meta-analysis. Gadolinium MRI Meta-analysis Group. Lancet 353:964-969
4. Filippi M (2001) In-vivo tissue characterization of multiple sclerosis and other white matter diseases using magnetic resonance based techniques. J Neurol 248 (*in press*)
5. De Stefano N, Matthews PM, Fu L et al (1998) Axonal damage correlates with disability in patients with relapsing-remitting multiple sclerosis. Results of a longitudinal magnetic resonance spectroscopy study. Brain 121:1469-1477
6. Fu L, Matthews PM, De Stefano N et al (1998) Imaging axonal damage of normal-appearing white matter in multiple sclerosis. Brain 121:103-113
7. Filippi M, Iannucci G, Tortorella C et al (1999) Comparison of MS clinical phenotypes using conventional and magnetization transfer MRI. Neurology 52:588-594
8. Filippi M, Bozzali M, Horsfield MA et al (2000) A conventional and magnetization transfer MRI study of the cervical cord in patients with MS. Neurology 54:207-213
9. Filippi M, Inglese M, Rovaris M et al (2000) Magnetization transfer imaging to monitor the evolution of MS: a 1-year follow-up study. Neurology 55:940-946
10. Tortorella C, Viti B, Bozzali M et al (2000) A magnetization transfer histogram study of normal-appearing brain tissue in MS. Neurology 54:186-193
11. Filippi M (2001) Linking structural, metabolic and functional changes in multiple sclerosis. Eur J Neurol 8:291-297

12. Mainero C, De Stefano N, Iannucci G et al (2001) Correlates of MS disability assessed in vivo using aggregates of MR quantities. Neurology 56:1331-1334
13. Ogawa S, Menon RS, Tank DW et al (1993) Functional brain mapping by blood oxygenation level-dependent contrast magnetic resonance imaging. A comparison of signal characteristics with a biophysical model. Biophys J 64:803-812
14. Jueptner M, Weiller C (1995) Review: does measurement of regional cerebral blood flow reflect synaptic activity? Implications for PET and fMRI. Neuroimage 2:148-156
15. Malonek D, Grinvald A (1996) Interactions between electrical activity and cortical microcirculation revealed by imaging spectroscopy: implications for functional brain mapping. Science 272:551-554
16. Vanzetta I, Grinvald A (1999) Increased cortical oxidative metabolism due to sensory stimulation: implications for functional brain imaging. Science 286:1555-1558
17. Ogawa S, Menon RS, Kim SG, Ugurbil K (1998) On the characteristics of functional magnetic resonance imaging of the brain. Annu Rev Biophys Biomol Struct 27:447-474
18. Bandettini PA, Jesmanowicz A, Wong EC, Hyde JS (1993) Processing strategies for time-course data sets in functional MRI of the human brain. Magn Reson Med 30:161-173
19. Rombouts SA, Lazeron RH, Scheltens P et al (1998) Visual activation patterns in patients with optic neuritis: an fMRI pilot study. Neurology 50:1896-1899
20. Werring DJ, Bullmore ET, Toosy AT et al (2000) Recovery from optic neuritis is associated with a change in the distribution of cerebral response to visual stimulation: a functional magnetic resonance imaging study. J Neurol Neurosurg Psychiatry 68:441-449
21. Clanet M, Berry I, Boulanouar K (1997) Functional imaging in multiple sclerosis. Int MS J 4:26-32
22. Lee M, Reddy H, Johansen-Berg H et al (2000) The motor cortex shows adaptive functional changes to brain injury from multiple sclerosis. Ann Neurol 47:606-613
23. Reddy H, Narayanan S, Arnoutelis R et al (2000) Evidence for adaptive functional changes in the cerebral cortex with axonal injury from multiple sclerosis. Brain 123:2314-2320
24. Reddy H, Narayanan S, Matthews PM et al (2000) Relating axonal injury to functional recovery in MS. Neurology 54:236-239
25. Rocca MA, Falini A, Colombo B et al (2002) Adaptive functional changes in the cerebral cortex of patients with non-disabling MS correlate with the extent of brain structural damage. Ann Neurol (*in press*)
26. Mesulam MM (1998) From sensation to cognition. Brain 121:1013-1052
27. Ferguson B, Matyszak MK, Esiri MM, Perry VH (1997) Axonal damage in acute multiple sclerosis lesions. Brain 120:393-399
28. Trapp BD, Ransohoff R, Rudick R (1999) Axonal pathology in multiple sclerosis: relationship to neurologic disability. Curr Opin Neurol 12:295-302
29. Brex PA, O'Riordan JI, Miszkiel KA et al (1999) Multisequence MRI in clinically isolated syndromes and the early development of MS. Neurology 53:1184-1190
30. Iannucci G, Tortorella C, Rovaris M et al (2000) Prognostic value of MR and magnetization transfer imaging findings in patients with clinically isolated syndromes suggestive of multiple sclerosis at presentation. AJNR Am J Neuroradiol 21:1034-1038
31. De Stefano N, Narayanan S, Francis GS et al (2001) Evidence of axonal damage in the early stages of multiple sclerosis and its relevance to disability. Arch Neurol 58:65-70
32. Cercignani M, Inglese M, Pagani E et al (2001) Mean diffusivity and fractional anisotropy histograms of patients with multiple sclerosis. AJNR Am J Neuroradiol 22:952-958
33. Waxman SG, Ritchie JM (1993) Molecular dissection of the myelinated axon. Ann Neurol 33:121-136
34. Lassmann H, Bruck W, Lucchinetti C, Rodriguez M (1997) Remyelination in multiple sclerosis. Mult Scler 3:133-136

35. De Stefano N, Narayanan S, Matthews PM et al (1999) In vivo evidence for axonal dysfunction remote from focal cerebral demyelination of the type seen in multiple sclerosis. Brain 122:1933-1939
36. Simmons ML, Frondoza CG, Coyle JT (1991) Immunohistochemical localization of N-acetyl-aspartate with monoclonal antibodies. Neuroscience 45:37-45
37. Weiller C, Chollet F, Friston KJ et al (1992) Functional reorganization of the brain in recovery from striatocapsular infarction in man. Ann Neurol 3:463-472
38. Chollet F, Weiller C (1994) Imaging recovery of function following brain injury. Curr Opin Neurobiol 4:226-230
39. Cramer SC, Nelles G, Benson RR et al (1997) A functional MRI study of subjects recovered from hemiparetic stroke. Stroke 28:2518-2527
40. Seil FJ (1997) Recovery and repair issues after stroke from the scientific perspective. Curr Opin Neurol 10:49-51
41. Cao Y, D'Olhaberriague L, Vikingstad EM et al (1998) Pilot study of functional MRI to assess cerebral activation of motor function after poststroke hemiparesis. Stroke 29:112-212
42. Thompson AJ, Montalban X, Barkhof F et al (2000) Diagnostic criteria for primary progressive multiple sclerosis: a position paper. Ann Neurol 47:831-835
43. Thompson AJ, Kermode AG, Wicks D et al (1991) Major differences in the dynamics of primary and secondary progressive multiple sclerosis. Ann Neurol 29:53-62
44. Kidd D, Thorpe JW, Kendall BE et al (1996) MRI dynamics of brain and spinal cord in progressive multiple sclerosis. J Neurol Neurosurg Psychiatry 60:15-19
45. Stevenson VL, Miller DH, Rovaris M et al (1999) Primary and transitional progressive MS: a clinical and MRI cross-sectional study. Neurology 52:839-845
46. Stevenson VL, Miller DH, Leary SM et al (2000) One year follow up study of primary and transitional progressive multiple sclerosis. J Neurol Neurosurg Psychiatry 68:713-718
47. Leary SM, Davie CA, Parker GJ et al (1999) 1H magnetic resonance spectroscopy of normal appearing white matter in primary progressive multiple sclerosis. J Neurol 246:1023-1026
48. Leary SM, Silver NC, Stevenson VL et al (1999) Magnetisation transfer of normal appearing white matter in primary progressive multiple sclerosis. Mult Scler 5:313-316
49. Rovaris M, Bozzali M, Santuccio G et al (2000) Relative contributions of brain and cervical cord pathology to multiple sclerosis disability: a study with magnetisation transfer ratio histogram analysis. J Neurol Neurosurg Psychiatry 69:723-727
50. Filippi M, Cercignani M, Inglese M et al (2001) Diffusion tensor magnetic resonance imaging in multiple sclerosis. Neurology 56:304-311
51. Bozzali M, Cercignani M, Comi G, Filippi M (2001) Gray matter involvement in multiple sclerosis phenotypes: a diffusion tensor and magnetization transfer imaging study (abstract). Proc Intl Soc Mag Reson Med 9:95
52. Rao SM, Binder JR, Bandettini PA et al (1993) Functional magnetic resonance imaging of complex human movements. Neurology 43:2311-2318
53. Paus T, Petrides M, Evans AC, Meyer E (1993) Role of the human anterior cingulate cortex in the control of oculomotor, manual, and speech responses: a positron emission tomography study. J Neurophysiol 70:453-469
54. Jenkins IH, Brooks DJ, Nixon PD et al (1994) Motor sequence learning: a study with positron emission tomography. J Neurosci 14:3775-3790
55. de Gelder B (2000) Neuroscience. More to seeing than meets the eye. Science 289:1148-1149
56. van Waesberghe JH, Kamphorst W, De Groot CJ et al (1999) Axonal loss in multiple sclerosis lesions: magnetic resonance imaging insights into substrates of disability. Ann Neurol 46:747-754
57. Pierpaoli C, Jezzard P, Basser PJ et al (1996) Diffusion tensor MR imaging of the human brain. Radiology 201:637-648

Subject Index